T0137354

Understanding the Host Immune Response Against *Mycobacterium tuberculosis* Infection

Vishwanath Venketaraman

Editor

Understanding the Host Immune Response Against *Mycobacterium tuberculosis* Infection

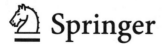 Springer

Editor
Vishwanath Venketaraman
Department of Basic Medical Sciences
Western University of Health Sciences
Pomona, CA, USA

ISBN 978-3-030-07344-2   ISBN 978-3-319-97367-8   (eBook)
https://doi.org/10.1007/978-3-319-97367-8

This Springer imprint is published by the registered company Springer Nature Switzerland AG
The registered company address is: Gewerbestrasse 11, 6330 Cham, Switzerland

Preface

According to the World Health Organization, approximately a third of the world population is latently infected with *Mycobacterium tuberculosis* (*M. tb* [LTBI]), with an estimated 9 million individuals with active tuberculosis (TB). It is estimated that approximately 2 million individuals die each year from active TB. In particular, 14.4% of these individuals have HIV and *M. tb* coinfection. Approximately 50–60% of these individuals with HIV and *M. tb* coinfection are from sub-Saharan Africa. HIV and *M. tb* coinfection continue to burden health-care systems in developing countries in both African and Asian subcontinent.

M. tb infection begins when individuals inhale infectious aerosol droplets containing *M. tb*. The inhaled bacilli are phagocytized by alveolar macrophages which are believed to provide the first line of defense against *M. tb* infection. TNF released by *M. tb*-infected macrophages is responsible for the formation and maintenance of granuloma, a critical immune response required to restrict and localize *M. tb* infection in the lungs, thereby preventing systemic dissemination of *M. tb* infection to other parts of the body.

Studies have shown that the T-helper 1 (Th1) subset of CD4+ T cell immunity plays an important role in augmenting the effector functions of macrophages to combating *M. tb* infection. It is believed that 90% of the healthy individuals mount an effective immune response against *M. tb* infection in the lungs, causing the bacteria to become dormant inside the granuloma, and this condition is referred to as LTBI.

M. tb is one of the leading causes of death in HIV-infected individuals. Chronic stages of HIV infection are usually accompanied by a progressive decline in the number of CD4+ T cells, which leads to disruption in the macrophage effector functions and weakened granulomatous responses against *M. tb* causing active TB. In HIV-TB coinfected individuals, *M. tb* can also systemically disseminate to other parts of the body to cause extrapulmonary TB. Recent evidence indicates that individuals with type 2 diabetes are increasingly susceptible to *M. tb* infection. Elderly individuals and chronic smokers are also at high risk for acquiring *M. tb* infection.

Understanding the effects of chronic conditions such as HIV, diabetes, chronic cigarette smoking, and aging, in dampening the immune responses will provide valuable information on the protective effector mechanisms that are key for defense against *M. tb* infection. This textbook provides a detailed review covering recent advances on topics such as:

1. Diabetes and TB
2. TB immunodiagnosis
3. Granulomatous responses to *Mycobacterium tuberculosis* infection
4. Animal models for tuberculosis
5. Host-directed therapies for tuberculosis
6. Cigarette smoking and increased susceptibility to tuberculosis
7. Coinfection with *Mycobacterium tuberculosis* and HIV

Pomona, CA, USA   Vishwanath Venketaraman

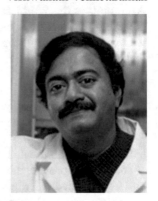

Contents

Contributors

John Brazil The Master's University, Santa Clarita, CA, USA

Caleb Cato Graduate College of Biomedical Sciences, Western University of Health Sciences, Pomona, CA, USA

Luke Elizabeth Hanna National Institute for Research in Tuberculosis, Chennai, India

Jennifer Hernandez Graduate College of Biomedical Sciences, Western University of Health Sciences, Pomona, CA, USA

Preet Kaur Graduate College of Biomedical Sciences, Western University of Health Sciences, Pomona, CA, USA

Imran H. Khan Department of Pathology and Laboratory Medicine, School of Medicine, University of California Davis Health System, Sacramento, CA, USA

Afsal Kolloli Public Health Research Institute, New Jersey Medical School at Rutgers Biomedical and Health Sciences, Rutgers University, Newark, NJ, USA

Jeff Koury Graduate College of Biomedical Sciences, Western University of Health Sciences, Pomona, CA, USA

Mariana Lucero Graduate College of Biomedical Sciences, Western University of Health Sciences, Pomona, CA, USA

Blanca I. Restrepo UTHealth Houston, School of Public Health, Brownsville, TX, USA

Pooja Singh Public Health Research Institute, New Jersey Medical School at Rutgers Biomedical and Health Sciences, Rutgers University, Newark, NJ, USA

Selvakumar Subbian Public Health Research Institute, New Jersey Medical School at Rutgers Biomedical and Health Sciences, Rutgers University, Newark, NJ, USA

Garrett Teskey Graduate College of Biomedical Sciences, Western University of Health Sciences, Pomona, CA, USA

Andrew Tran Graduate College of Biomedical Sciences, Western University of Health Sciences, Pomona, CA, USA

Vishwanath Venketaraman Graduate College of Biomedical Sciences, Western University of Health Sciences, Pomona, CA, USA

Department of Basic Medical Sciences, College of Osteopathic Medicine of the Pacific, Western University of Health Sciences, Pomona, CA, USA

Diabetes and Tuberculosis

Blanca I. Restrepo

Diabetes mellitus is characterized by hyperglycemia due to defects in insulin secretion, insulin response, or both (American-Diabetes-Association 2014). Type 1 and type 2 diabetes (T2D) patients have a higher morbidity and mortality from pulmonary infections, with tuberculosis (TB) being a prominent example (Muller et al. 2005; Shah and Hux 2003). In this chapter the focus is mostly on T2D which is the most prevalent form. The worldwide increase in the prevalence of T2D in low- and middle-income countries where TB is most endemic is a recognized reemerging risk and challenge to TB control (Ottmani et al. 2010). Individuals with T2D have three times the risk of developing TB, and there are now more individuals with TB-T2D comorbidity than TB-HIV coinfection (Jeon and Murray 2008; Ronacher et al. 2015). The frequent co-occurrence of diabetes (type 1 or type 2) and TB was first described centuries ago by the Persian philosopher Avincenna. The comorbidity was a frequent topic in the medical literature in the first half of the twentieth century, but its notoriety was reduced with the introduction of insulin treatment for type 1 diabetes and antibiotics for TB (Boucot et al. 1952; Morton 1694; Root 1934; Silwer and Oscarsson 1958). In the 1980s, the publications on joint TB-T2D began to reappear with the number of publications on TB and T2D rising exponentially in contemporary times as the global prevalence of T2D among adults has continued to rise (Fig. 1). Diabetes is predicted to reach 642 million worldwide by 2040 with most (80%) of the patients living in low- and middle-income countries where TB is also endemic (International-Diabetes-Federation 2015). The World Health Organization has identified T2D as a neglected, important, and reemerging risk factor for TB (Ottmani et al. 2010). In this chapter, "T2D" will refer mostly to type 2 diabetes since it is the most prevalent form, but type 1 diabetes in children has also been associated with TB (International-Diabetes-Federation 2015; Webb et al. 2009). This chapter

B. I. Restrepo (✉)
UTHealth Houston, School of Public Health, Brownsville, TX, USA
e-mail: blanca.i.restrepo@uth.tmc.edu

© Springer Nature Switzerland AG 2018   1
V. Venketaraman (ed.), *Understanding the Host Immune Response Against Mycobacterium tuberculosis Infection*, https://doi.org/10.1007/978-3-319-97367-8_1

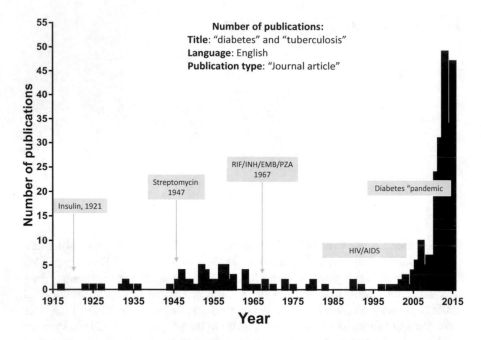

Fig. 1 Historical perspective of the association between TB and diabetes based on the number of publications. Most of the literature on the comorbidity was published between the 1940s and 1960s, but thereafter the topic lost notoriety with the improved control of type 1 diabetes with insulin and the implementation of antibiotics that could effectively cure most TB patients. In the 1980s, HIV emerged and continues to be the most notable risk factor for TB. But in contemporary times there have been improvements in HIV treatment and a notable increase in diabetes worldwide "pandemic," resulting in an exponential increase in the number of publications on the topic

provides an overview of the epidemiology of TB-T2D, the impact of T2D on the clinical presentation and outcomes of TB, and the underlying biology that favors the co-occurrence of both diseases.

Epidemiology

Risk of TB development among TB patients. Obesity has increased worldwide due to population aging, urbanization and reduced physical activity, resulting in an increasing prevalence of type 2 diabetes (Hu 2011). About 80% of the 415 million estimated T2D cases globally are from low- and middle-income countries, and its prevalence is projected to continue rising over the next 30 years, particularly in regions with high TB incidence (International-Diabetes-Federation 2015) (Fig. 2). It is well accepted that T2D increases the risk of TB. A recent systematic review and meta-analysis of 44 studies found that T2D increases the risk of TB by two- to four-fold (Al-Rifai et al. 2017). There is wide variation between studies worldwide with

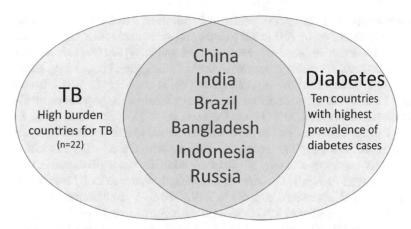

Fig. 2 Convergence of countries with highest burden of TB and T2D worldwide. Among the 10 countries with the highest number of diabetes patients worldwide, 6 are also among the 22 high-burden countries that contribute 80% of the TB cases worldwide. (Updated from Restrepo (2007))

risk ratios ranging between 0.99 and 7.83. This illustrates the complexity of studying T2D as a risk factor for TB given the heterogeneity in T2D populations worldwide, methods for T2D diagnosis which range from self-reported (least sensitive) to oral glucose tolerance test (more sensitive), and also in study designs (Kornfeld et al. 2016). These risk ratios can be affected by the T2D patient's age, access to healthcare, level of glucose control, and T2D complications and medications. For example, the co-occurrence of T2D with other host characteristics can synergize to increase TB risk among T2D patients, as suggested for T2D plus smoking, micro- and macro-vascular complications of T2D, host metabolism, and even the social environment (Kuo et al. 2013; Lonnroth et al. 2009; Reed et al. 2013). Differences in the risk ratios are also observed between study designs (Al-Rifai et al. 2017; Huangfu et al. 2017). This heterogeneity calls for the need for study designs that include a thorough characterization of T2D and other host factors, and with multi-variable analysis in order to reach conclusions that are comparable between studies.

As studies on the epidemiology of TB-T2D increase worldwide, certain regions display particularly high prevalence rates of T2D among TB, including South India (54%), the Pacific Islands (40%), and northeastern Mexico (36%) (Kornfeld et al. 2016; Restrepo et al. 2011; Restrepo et al. 2007; Viney et al. 2014). However, developed countries can have subpopulations with similar hotspots, as is the case of US communities adjacent to Mexico where the T2D prevalence among TB patients is nearly 40% (Restrepo et al. 2011). The co-occurrence of TB-T2D is projected to continue increasing: A longitudinal analysis of 163 countries reported a parallel increase in TB incidence and T2D prevalence (Goldhaber-Fiebert et al. 2011). In Mexico, longitudinal analysis reported increases in the prevalence of TB-T2D among TB patients over an 8- or 12-year period of time of 2.8% and 83%, respectively (Abdelbary et al. 2016; Delgado-Sanchez et al. 2015).

Contribution of T2D to TB control: Population attributable fraction. The reported contribution of T2D to TB (population attributable fraction) was estimated to be 13% worldwide (generally between 10% and 20%) but can vary substantially (Lonnroth et al. 2014). For example, in the UK, the general population attributable risk is 10%, but rises to 20% in Asian males (Walker and Unwin 2010). In countries where TB and T2D are endemic such as India or Mexico, the population attributable fraction reaches at least 20% (Ponce-De-Leon et al. 2004; Stevenson et al. 2007b). In the Texas-Mexico border, the population attributable fraction is 28% for all adult TB cases, but rises to 51% among TB patients who are 35–60 years old. In this region, HIV contributes to only 3–6% of the adult TB cases (Restrepo et al. 2011). Therefore, even though T2D confers a significantly lower risk of TB at the individual level (threefold) when compared to HIV (>20-fold), in communities like these where the sheer number of T2D patients is high, the contribution of T2D to TB can be higher than HIV (Getahun et al. 2010). A study using dynamic TB transmission models to analyze the potential effects of T2D on TB epidemiology in 13 countries with high burden of TB concluded that stopping the rise of T2D would avoid 6 million (95% CI 5.1, 6.9) incident cases and 1.1 million (1.0, 1.3) TB deaths in these countries in 20 years (Pan et al. 2015). Thus, every community worldwide needs to evaluate the prevalence of T2D and its contribution to TB. This information is variable between regions and critical to guide for the most efficient use of limited resources for TB control programs.

T2D versus transient hyperglycemia. Most studies on TB-T2D are observational with few cohorts available from countries that have nationwide health information systems that permit studies with 100,000s of participants (Al-Rifai et al. 2017; Restrepo and Schlesinger 2014). All cohorts to date indicate that T2D develops before TB, and those with further characterization of the T2D patients suggest that it is not T2D in itself, but rather poorly controlled T2D that increases TB risk (Baker et al. 2012; Kuo et al. 2013; Leung et al. 2008). Cross-sectional studies also support the concept of T2D preceding TB, with chronic T2D patients (median 7 years) that present other T2D complications prior to TB development (Abdelbary et al. 2016; Restrepo et al. 2011; Stevenson et al. 2007a). This highlights the missed opportunities for preventing TB among T2D patients who have presumably been in contact for years with their healthcare providers. However, TB-T2D patients should be distinguished from TB patients with transient hyperglycemia secondary to the inflammation induced during TB (Boillat-Blanco et al. 2016). The distinction between T2D and transient hyperglycemia can be established once the TB patient is no longer febrile. Nevertheless, assessment of hyperglycemia at the time of TB diagnosis, whether it is T2D or transient hyperglycemia, can be helpful to detect patients at risk for adverse outcomes (Boillat-Blanco et al. 2016).

Contribution of TB and T2D on new T2D diagnosis. It is estimated half of the patients with T2D in developing countries are not aware of their T2D diagnosis. The higher risk of T2D among TB patients has expanded the role of TB clinics as hubs for new diagnosis of T2D worldwide, with high variations in T2D awareness between countries (2% in south Texas, USA, and up to 37% in Chennai, India) (Kornfeld et al. 2016; Restrepo et al. 2011). Most importantly, the newly diagnosed T2D patients with TB (versus previously diagnosed T2D) have a different profile: they are more likely to be males, younger patients, and with lower HbA1cs (Abdelbary et al. 2016; Kornfeld et al. 2016; Restrepo et al. 2011). This highlights the importance of TB clinics to reach males who are not as likely to be in contact with the healthcare system when compared to females, or to identify patients who are at an earlier stage of their T2D before the presentation of additional and irreversible micro- and macro-vascular complications of T2D. As more T2D patients are diagnosed, the next public health challenge for low- and middle-income countries where both diseases are most likely to converge is to provide immediate attention to TB treatment, but also the long-term care required for T2D in order to avoid its chronic and life-threatening complications.

Clinical Aspects

Nearly all studies comparing the clinical presentation of TB-T2D patients versus TB-no T2D find that those with T2D comorbidity are more likely to present with pulmonary (versus extrapulmonary), cavitary (versus noncavitary), and sputum smear-positive TB at diagnosis. Furthermore, during TB treatment the TB-T2D patients take longer to convert from sputum smear-positive to smear-negative. Some studies, but not others, find that TB-T2D patients are more likely to present with drug-resistant and multidrug resistant TB (Fig. 3).

Pulmonary versus extra-pulmonary TB. About 70–80% of the TB patients have pulmonary TB, with the remaining proportion presenting only extrapulmonary

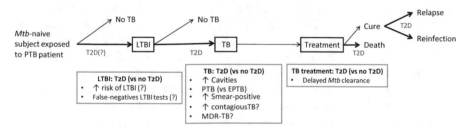

Fig. 3 Role of T2D on the development and treatment of TB. *M. tuberculosis*-naïve individuals who have T2D have a threefold higher risk of TB. This may be primary or reactivation TB. T2D patients may also be more likely to develop or persist with latent TB infection (LTBI), although this is not confirmed ("?"). The TB-T2D host is more likely to present with clinical characteristics associated with enhanced TB transmission, but the impact of disease spread in the community has not been systematically studied (bottom text box; "T2D?"). TB treatment outcomes include cure, treatment failure, or death. T2D increases the risk of failure or death. Among presumably cured individuals TB relapses may also be more likely to occur. PTB pulmonary TB, EPTB extrapulmonary TB, LTBI latent TB infection

involvement that is usually attributed to immune compromise that allows hematogenous dissemination of *M. tuberculosis*. This is the case for TB patients with HIV-AIDS (Leeds et al. 2012) or taking TNF blockers (Harris and Keane 2010). In contrast, TB-T2D patients are less likely to present with extrapulmonary TB (Leung et al. 2008; Reis-Santos et al. 2013; Restrepo et al. 2007; Viswanathan et al. 2012). A possible explanation is that T2D is characterized by a dysfunctional immune response with hyper-reactive cell-mediated response to *M. tuberculosis*. This cell-mediated response may be suboptimal for containing *M. tuberculosis* growth within the lung but effective for preventing its dissemination to the periphery (Kumar et al. 2013b; Restrepo et al. 2008a; Walsh et al. 2010). Another possible explanation is a compromised sentinel function in alveolar macrophages, but not peripheral macrophages, in diabetes (Martinez et al. 2016).

Cavitary and smear-positive TB. TB-T2D patients are more likely than TB-no T2D to present with smear- positive and cavitary TB. Both observations are related. The cell-mediated response induced by *M. tuberculosis* results in the formation of pulmonary granulomas (tubercles) that are thought to be a double- edged sword for the host (Guirado et al. 2013). Granulomas initially limit *M. tuberculosis* growth, but in hosts in whom *M. tuberculosis* continues to replicate, these structures undergo central caseation with rupturing and spilling of thousands of viable bacilli into the airways. This "cavitary TB" is associated with sputum smear- positivity (Restrepo 2007; Russell 2007; Viswanathan et al. 2012). The high bacillary burden (based on higher positive smears) in TB-T2D patients at the time of TB diagnosis is consistent with their delayed smear conversion from positive to negative (Perez-Navarro et al. 2017; Restrepo et al. 2008b; Viswanathan et al. 2014). The combination of higher PTB, cavitary TB, and smear-positive TB at diagnosis and during treatment predicts that TB-T2D patients are more infectious and for a longer period of time, than TB-no T2D (Behr et al. 1999). If confirmed, this would be yet another public health implication for the TB-T2D comorbidity.

Drug and multidrug resistant (MDR) TB. The relationship between drug-resistant and MDR TB in T2D is unclear and with conflicting results between studies (Abdelbary et al. 2016; Bashar et al. 2001; Fisher-Hoch et al. 2008; Gomez-Gomez et al. 2015; Hsu et al. 2013; Magee et al. 2013; Magee et al. 2015; Perez-Navarro et al. 2015; Subhash et al. 2003; Wang and Lin 2001). In a meta-analysis, the prevalence of drug-resistant or MDR TB among recurrent TB cases was not significantly higher in TB-T2D patients (OR 1.24, 95% CI 0.72, 2.16) (Baker et al. 2011). However, these findings are based on only four studies and a limitation is that most of the countries with a high incidence of TB only do DR testing after the initial empiric treatment with first-line drugs fail (Abdelbary et al. 2017). Therefore, appropriate testing for MDR TB among the entire population at the time of TB diagnosis (not just those with treatment failures) is required in order to understand the circumstances under which MDR TB and T2D may synergize.

TB Treatment Outcomes in TB-T2D Patients

Some observational studies have reported an association between TB-T2D and adverse TB treatment outcomes, including delays in mycobacterial clearance, treatment failures, death, relapse, and reinfection (Fig. 4) (Baker et al. 2012; Jeon et al. 2012; Jimenez-Corona et al. 2013)

Delays in sputum smear clearance and treatment failure. TB-T2D versus TB-no T2D patients are more likely to remain sputum smear-positive after completion of the intensive phase of treatment, and this outcome is an early predictor of treatment failure (sputum smear or culture positivity at 5 months or later during treatment), which is also more likely in TB-T2D versus TB-no T2D (Baker et al. 2011; Jimenez-Corona et al. 2013; Viswanathan et al. 2014).

Death. In a systematic review and meta-analysis of contemporary literature, Baker et al. concluded that the risk of death from TB or any other cause in 23 unadjusted studies was nearly twofold (RR 1.89; 95% CI 1.52–2.36), and this increased to 4.95 (95% CI 2.69–9.10) in 4 studies that adjusted for age and potential confounders (Baker et al. 2011). But not all studies find an increased risk of death in T2D patients (Abdelbary et al. 2017; Jimenez-Corona et al. 2013; Viswanathan et al. 2014). It has been suggested that death in TB-T2D may be from complications of T2D, and not necessarily from TB (Prada-Medina et al. 2017; Reed et al. 2013), even though transient hyperglycemia at the time of TB diagnosis has been shown to predict treatment failure and death in patients from Tanzania (Boillat-Blanco et al. 2016).

Relapse and reinfection. TB-T2D patients also appear to have a higher risk of relapse. The review by Baker et al. reported a nearly fourfold risk of relapse in TB-T2D versus TB-no T2D (RR 3.89; 95% CI 2.43–6.23) (Baker et al. 2011). A prospective study in southern Mexico with 1262 TB patients characterized for

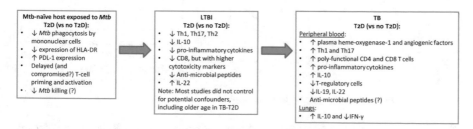

Fig. 4 Dysfunctional immunity in T2D hosts at different stages of the natural history of TB. As the natural history of TB evolves in the T2D host, so does the immune response with characteristics that contrast with the non-T2D host. The *M. tuberculosis*-naïve hosts have a delayed and underperforming innate response. The level of responsiveness of the pro-inflammatory or anti-inflammatory immune response is also lower in individuals with LTBI, although many of these studies did not control for confounders, including the older age of the T2D patients compared to no T2D. Once the TB patient develops T2D, there is an "exaggerated" response in peripheral blood, but this may be tampered in the lungs. Details are provided in the text

M. tuberculosis genotypes further distinguished between relapses and reinfections and found higher adjusted odds of both outcomes in T2D versus no T2D (OR = 1.8 for both recurrence and relapse) (Jimenez-Corona et al. 2013).

Underlying Biology for the Association Between TB and T2D

The most plausible link between T2D and TB is the presence of a dysfunctional (not necessarily immunocompromised) immune response that is ineffective for clearing Mtb. The most likely underlying mechanism is chronic hyperglycemia (poorly controlled glucose with high HbA1c) and its metabolic consequences, which include the deleterious accumulation of reactive oxidative species (ROS) (Fig. 5) (Lagman et al. 2015). The chronic upregulation of glucose can lead to the abnormal accumulation of glucose intermediates and to excessive reactive oxidative species via different pathways. These include advanced glycation end products (AGE) like methyl

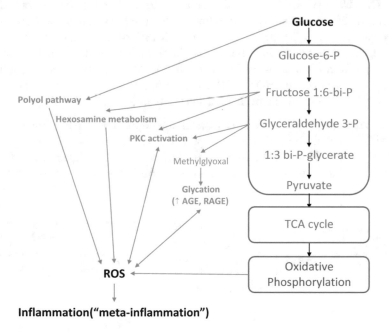

Fig. 5 Diabetes is associated with accumulation of glycolysis intermediates that favor oxidation and inflammation. Hyperglycemia is associated with the accumulation of glycolysis intermediates that lead to increase in various pathways: (i) polyol pathway, (ii) formation of AGEs and upregulation of its receptor, RAGE, (iii) activation of protein kinase C isoforms, and (iv) increased hexosamine pathway. These pathways, as well as the overproduction of reactive oxidative species (ROS) in the mitochondria, favor the formation or accumulation of ROS, which further increases the occurrence of these pathways. The overproduction of ROS is believed to be the underlying mechanism for T2D complications, including the chronic inflammation and vascular complications characteristic of these patients. These pathways are also likely to underlie the dysfunctional immunity to *M. tuberculosis*, and hence, the higher susceptibility of its patients to TB

glycoxal are highly reactive and can bind and modify immune response molecules (e.g., antibodies, complement), although the impact on function is still unclear (Goetze et al. 2012; Stirban et al. 2014). Excess AGE may also promote constant stimulation of its scavenger receptor, RAGE, leading to aberrant stimulation of phagocytes with activation of NFκB and NADPH oxidase (Brownlee 2001). Excessive NADPH activity leads to the accumulation of reactive oxidative species and contributes to oxidative stress. The excessive accumulation of glucose intermediates also leads to uncoupling of the oxidative phosphorylation reactions in the mitochondria, which result in excessive generation of superoxide anion and downstream reactive oxidative species, further contributing to the oxidative status that characterizes patients with diabetes (Giacco and Brownlee 2010). A summary of the key innate and adaptive components of the immune response to *M. tuberculosis* is provided elsewhere in this book, and in this chapter we focus on the description of altered responses in the host with T2D.

Immune Response Studies in TB-Naïve Hosts with T2D

The early events after inhalation of *M. tuberculosis* by a TB-naive host are critical determinants of disease outcome. Innate immunity is incapable of restricting bacillary replication but plays a pivotal role in activating the adaptive response that controls infection. Recapitulation of these early events is not possible in humans, so data is based on in vitro studies with TB-naïve hosts or evaluation of the initial events following *M. tuberculosis* infection in animal models of TB-T2D.

The macrophage system includes circulating monocytes, tissue macrophages (alveolar macrophages in the lungs), and dendritic cells. In the T2D host, studies unrelated to TB indicate these phagocytic cells have impaired phagocytic, chemotactic, and bactericidal capacity and have an altered phenotype (Fernandez-Real and Pickup 2012; Pickup 2004). A few studies in TB-naïve humans are beginning to show a similar phenotype when challenged with *M. tuberculosis*. Most studies find that monocytes or monocyte-derived macrophages from healthy individuals with poorly controlled T2D (versus non-T2D or T2D with good glucose control) have significantly reduced association (binding and phagocytosis) of *M. tuberculosis* (Gomez et al. 2013; Lopez-Lopez et al. 2018). We find that this defect appears to be attributed to alterations in the diabetic monocyte itself as well as in serum opsonins for *M. tuberculosis*, particularly the C3 component of complement which mediates *M. tuberculosis* phagocytosis (Gomez et al. 2013; Restrepo et al. 2014). Lopez-Lopez and collaborators find that the lower phagocytosis of diabetic MT2Ds is dependent on the use of more virulent strains of *M. tuberculosis* (Lopez-Lopez et al. 2018). Another study (LTBI status not indicated) reported that the monocytes from participants with T2D and deficient serum vitamin D (but not T2D alone), allowed for higher *M. tuberculosis* growth. This reduced capacity for *M. tuberculosis* growth containment was associated with diminished nitric oxide production and not with antimicrobial peptide expression (Herrera et al. 2017). Studies in diabetic mice confirm the findings in humans. Murine alveolar macrophages also have a reduced uptake of *M. tuberculosis* in the first 2 weeks of infection (Martinez et al. 2016; Martinez and Kornfeld 2014). This reduced phagocytosis has been associated with diminished expression of cell surface receptors (CD14, MARCO) and is unique to alveolar macrophages (versus peritoneal or bone-marrow derived macrophages). This reduced sentinel function results in the late delivery of *M. tuberculosis* by antigen- presenting cells to the lung draining lymph nodes and delayed initiation of cell-mediated immunity, resulting in higher *M. tuberculosis* burden as the infection progresses (Vallerskog et al. 2010). Together, the findings in diabetic humans and mice indicate an under-performing innate immune response during the initial encounter with *M. tuberculosis*. Since the efficient phagocytosis and priming of the adaptive immune responses are necessary to activate the cell-mediated immune response that restricts initial *M. tuberculosis* growth (Vallerskog et al. 2010), these delays are postulated to contribute to the higher risk of T2D patients for *M. tuberculosis* infection and persistence (Fig. 3).

Immune Response Studies in Individuals with LTBI and T2D

There is growing literature for studies in individuals with LTBI and T2D (LTBI-T2D) versus LTBI-no T2D, with a summary provided in Fig. 3. Most studies have been done in Chennai, India, and suggest that at baseline there are diminished frequencies of TB-specific pro-inflammatory (Th1 and Th17) and anti-inflammatory (IL-10 and Th2) cells (Kumar et al. 2014; Kumar et al. 2016a). The in vitro stimulation of CD4-positive cells with mycobacterial antigens also results in lower secretion of pro- and anti-inflammatory cytokines. A similar observation is reported for CD8-positive T cells, but curiously, these cells have increased expression of cytotoxic markers in LTBI-T2D (Kumar et al. 2016b). In studies using whole blood, the addition of neutralizing antibodies to IL-10 and TGF-β abrogated the difference between LTBI by T2D status (Kumar et al. 2016a). A study in Mexico reported lower expression of antimicrobial peptides, specifically Cathelicidin LL-37, Defensin A-1, and Defensin B-4 in LTBI-T2D (Gonzalez-Curiel et al. 2011). Thus, the studies in India and Mexico suggest lower levels of pro-inflammatory responses that could favor the progression from LTBI to TB in diabetic patients. A study in Tanzania, Africa, among healthy controls (neighborhood controls to TB patients) reported that those with T2D (vs non-T2D) had a lower proportion of QFT-positives and lower levels of IFN-γ secreted in response to mycobacterial antigens. However, after adjusting for confounders the differences between study groups did not reach significance (Faurholt-Jepsen et al. 2014). Of note, in the studies in India and Mexico the participants with T2D were older and had difference in dyslipidemias when compared to no T2D, but there was no reporting of the adjusted estimates. Together, these studies suggest that lower levels of pro-inflammatory cytokines in T2D can favor progression from LTBI to TB in T2D, but further studies are required to understand the impact of lower anti-inflammatory cytokines as well, and the potential confounding effect of age and dylipidemias to these findings.

Immune Response Studies in Individuals with TB and T2D

Most of the immunological studies assessing the association between TB and T2D have compared TB patients with T2D (TB-T2D), versus no T2D (TB-no T2D) with a summary provided in Fig. 3. Baseline (plasma) levels of cytokines are higher in TB-T2D (vs TB-no T2D), including Th1 (IFN-ɣ, TNFa, IL-2), Th17 (IL-17A), Type 2 (IL-5), pro- inflammatory (IL-1b, IL-6, IL-18), and anti-inflammatory (IL-10) (Kumar et al. 2013a). Plasma levels of TB-T2D patients are also characterized by heightened levels of heme oxygenase-1, an indicator of oxidative stress, and of angiogenic factors (VEGF-A, C, D) and its soluble receptors (VEGF-R1, R2, and R3) (Andrade et al. 2014; Kumar et al. 2017a). Antimicrobial peptides are reportedly higher, lower, or similar by T2D status, depending on the study (Gonzalez-Curiel et al. 2011; Kumar et al. 2017b; Zhan and Jiang 2015). Thus, baseline levels of cytokines in T2D and pre-T2D are characterized by a balanced upregulation of pro- and anti-inflammatory cytokines. An exception is the IL-20 family of cytokines, notably IL-19 and IL-22, which have lower expression (Kumar et al. 2015a). This is interesting given the beneficial metabolic effects of IL-22 (Dalmas and Donath 2014; Hasnain et al. 2014).

The response of blood cells from TB-T2D to *M. tuberculosis* antigens in vitro is also characterized by a hyper-inflammatory response in most studies. Namely, stimulation of cells in whole blood or peripheral blood mononuclear cells (PBMCs) with mycobacterial antigens results in higher Th1 and Th17 responses (except IL-22), including higher IFN-ɣ, IL-2, GM-CSF, and IL-17 secretion (Kumar et al. 2013b; Restrepo et al. 2008a; Walsh et al. 2010) (Fig. 6 for IL-2 and IFN- ɣ). TB-T2D cases also have a higher frequency of single- and double-cytokine producing CD4+ Th1 cells in response to *M. tuberculosis* antigens (for IFN-ɣ, TNF-α, or IL-2) (Kumar et al. 2013b). There is also expansion of CD8 T cells and NK cells (Kumar et al. 2015b). However, some studies report apparently different results. In Indonesia or Tanzania, researchers found no differences in IFN-ɣ responses to mycobacterial antigens in TB patients by T2D status (Stalenhoef et al. 2008; Blanco-Boillat in press). Furthermore, in Tanzania the researchers found that IFN-ɣ secretion by CD4+ T cells was lower in TB- T2D versus TB-no T2D in response to the nonvirulent vaccine strain, *M. bovis* BCG. While they conclude that the lower Th1 response to the live bacteria versus the purified antigens (ESAT-6 and CFP-10) was due to the need for antigen processing in the former, but not the later, it is also possible that this difference is attributed to other experimental factors such as the absence of ESAT-6 and CFP-10 in *M. bovis* BCG, which are virulence factors known to affect immune responses in *M. tuberculosis*. Accordingly, in TB-naive hosts with T2D, Lopez- Lopez found differences in the response of diabetic MT2Ds that appeared to vary by *M. tuberculosis* virulence status, although sample size was small in this study (Lopez-Lopez et al. 2018).There are some distinctive feature of the study from Tanzania versus the other studies that could also contribute to reduced IFN-ɣ secretion in the former study: (i) T2D classification was carefully done by excluding anyone with transient hyperglycemia detected at the time of TB diagnosis,

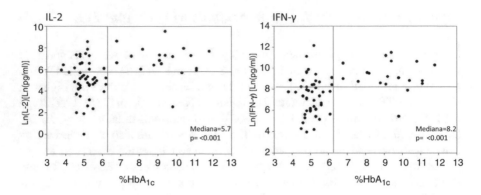

Fig. 6 Higher IFN-γ secretion in response to PPD in TB patients with high HbA1c (versus normal HbA1c) despite their T2D status. Whole blood from TB patients +/− T2D was incubated with purified protein derivative (PPD) from *M. tuberculosis* and after 18–24 h the secretion of IFN-γ was quantified by ELISA in the culture supernatants. Results are shown in scatter plots where each circle represents one TB patient. The horizontal line indicates the median IFN-γ level. The vertical line at the HbA1c level of 6.2% of total hemoglobin indicates the upper limits of normal *(left)* and elevated *(right)* HbA1c level. IFN-γ values are provided in natural log (Ln) scale. (Adapted from Restrepo et al. (2008a))

(ii) most of the T2D patients were taking hypoglycemic agents or insulin (despite this they still had poor glucose control), (iii) their algorithm for assessment of IFN-γ secretion by flow cytometry subtracted any background cytokine levels, (iv) they used frozen (vs fresh) PBMCs for the experiments, and (v) their sample size was small and included TB-T2D and LTBI-T2D participants. These variations in results reinforce the importance of additional studies to understand the role played by individual hosts and experimental factors that influence the differential responses in the patients with T2D.

Studies in Individuals with TB and T2D Using Alveolar Macro phages

The hyperactive responses in peripheral blood contrast with the results from few studies conducted at the site of infection (in bronchoalveolar lavage) where TB-T2D patients appear to have reduced activation of immunity; one reported a lower proportion of activated alveolar macrophages (Wang et al. 1999), and another higher anti-inflammatory (IL-10) and lower pro-inflammatory (IFN-γ) cytokines (Sun et al. 2012). The impact of the host compartment (peripheral blood versus lung) requires further study. In diabetic mice, a reduction in *M. tuberculosis* phagocytosis is only observed in alveolar macrophages, but not resting peritoneal or bone marrow-derived macrophages (Martinez et al. 2016). However, as *M. tuberculosis* replicates in these mice, there is higher pulmonary *M. tuberculosis* burden and more extensive inflammation with higher expression of pro-inflammatory cytokines like IFN-γ in the lungs (Cheekatla et al. 2016; Martens et al. 2007; Vallerskog et al. 2010; Yamashiro et al. 2005). These findings in the lungs of mice resemble the hyper-response to *M. tuberculosis* antigens in the peripheral blood of TB-T2D (versus TB-no T2D) patients, with similar findings in the guinea pig model of TB-T2D (Podell et al. 2014).

Together, most of the studies in TB-T2D hosts suggest a normal or even exaggerated pro-inflammatory response, when compared to no T2D, but further studies are needed to understand observed differences between studies. There are several possible explanations for the contribution of dysfunctional immunity to these adverse treatment outcomes. (1) The higher Th1 and Th17 response is only present in the peripheral blood of TB-T2D patients, while anti-inflammatory responses that facilitate *M. tuberculosis* growth only occur in the lungs. (2) There is a higher production of pro-inflammatory cytokines like IFN-γ in the lungs of humans (as observed in mice), but it is not effective for downstream activation of macrophages or cytotoxic T cells that ultimately kill *M. tuberculosis*. (3) The hyper-reaction to *M. tuberculosis* antigens may be deleterious and contribute to lung tissue damage with more severe TB and the higher frequency of death in TB-T2D patients. (4) The inflammatory response in T2D is suitable for controlling *M. tuberculosis*, and the higher risk of TB in the T2D host is mostly imparted by a delayed or inefficient early innate response. These possibilities are not mutually exclusive and understanding the complex balance in the timing, type, and intensity of the response in TB-T2D will help improve the clinical management of TB patients.

Host-Directed Therapies for TB in T2D Patients

Current TB research interests include the identification of host-directed therapies that synergize with antibiotics for effective *M. tuberculosis* elimination. The goal of these host-directed therapies is to boost immune mechanisms that diminish excess inflammation to reduce lung tissue damage and limit *M. tuberculosis* growth. Coincidently, the most common medication for type 2 diabetes, metformin, is one of the candidates for TB host-directed therapy (Zumla et al. 2015). Preliminary findings suggest metformin may be beneficial for TB control by reducing the deleterious inflammation associated with immune pathology and enhancing the anti-mycobacterial activity of immune cells (Singhal et al. 2014). Additional studies are now required to further elucidate the underlying relationship between metformin and *M. tuberculosis* killing, with careful assessment of the risks involved by adding anti-inflammatory medications like metformin to the TB regimen (Restrepo 2016).

T2D patients are also characterized by dyslipidemia, and another candidate drug for host-directed therapy are statins, which lower cholesterol and may contribute to *M. tuberculosis* containment by diminishing the formation of lipid bodies inside *M. tuberculosis*-infected macrophages (and additional effects of statins on immunity) (Lai et al. 2016; Parihar et al. 2014; Su et al. 2017).

Finally, T2D and TB patients are also characterized by higher oxidative stress (Fig. 4), and in one study this was associated with reduced expression of IL-12, a key cytokine for promoting Th1 responses to *M. tuberculosis* (Tan et al. 2012). Consistent with these findings, the aT2Dinistration of reduced glutathione in liposomal presentation appears to be effective in vitro for decreasing the survival and intracellular growth of *M. tuberculosis*. Liposomal GSH also decreased the over expressed levels of pro-inflammatory cytokines secreted from in vitro generated granulomas from individuals with T2D (Islamoglu et al. 2018). A clinical trial to evaluate the effectiveness of liposomal GSH is currently underway (Venketaraman, personal communication).

Concluding Remarks

The higher prevalence of T2D in low- and middle-income countries where TB is endemic has been identified as one of the factors that will hinder the global TB target of 90% reduction in TB incidence by 2035 (Odone et al. 2014). Several challenges need to be addressed: How can we prevent the development of TB among T2D patients? This will require the stratification of the millions of T2D patients who have LTBI, into those who have higher TB risk. Such stratification will require the combination of clinical, epidemiological, and immunological markers in order to develop models for tailored and cost-effective recommendations for LTBI treatment. Glucose control appears to be a major factor associated with TB risk and adverse TB treatment outcomes in the clinical setting (Jorgensen and Faurholt-Jepsen 2014), and with altered immunity in the basic science studies. Glucose control is also the mainstay for the prevention of other T2D complications (DCCTRG et al. 1993).

However, other conditions associated with T2D, such as dyslipidemias, or the presence of other known risk factors for TB unrelated to T2D, such as smoking, are likely to be important and have been poorly characterized on T2D patients. Furthermore, the apparently simple goal of achieving good glucose control among T2D patients, particularly in low- and middle-income countries, is a major challenge that will require a multidisciplinary approach. Epidemiological, clinical, and basic science research should guide the identification of simple and measurable risk factors for TB development at the individual level, and the public health and healthcare systems should make policy and adopt these findings. Only then will we be able to stratify TB risk with more precision for targeted TB prevention among the millions of T2D patients at risk for TB.

References

Abdelbary, B. E., Garcia-Viveros, M., Ramirez-Oropesa, H., Rahbar, M. H., & Restrepo, B. I. (2016). Tuberculosis-diabetes epidemiology in the border and non-border regions of Tamaulipas, Mexico. *Tuberculosis (Edinburgh, Scotland), 101S*, S124–S134.

Abdelbary, B. E., Garcia-Viveros, M., Ramirez-Oropesa, H., Rahbar, M. H., & Restrepo, B. I. (2017). Predicting treatment failure, death and drug resistance using a computed risk score among newly diagnosed TB patients in Tamaulipas, Mexico. *Epidemiology and Infection, 145*, 3020–3034.

Al-Rifai, R. H., Pearson, F., Critchley, J. A., & Abu-Raddad, L. J. (2017). Association between diabetes mellitus and active tuberculosis: A systematic review and meta-analysis. *PLoS One, 12*, e0187967.

American-Diabetes-Association. (2014). Standards of medical care in diabetes--2014. *Diabetes Care, 37*(Suppl 1), S14–S80.

Andrade, B. B., Pavan, K. N., Sridhar, R., Banurekha, V. V., Jawahar, M. S., Nutman, T. B., Sher, A., & Babu, S. (2014). Heightened plasma levels of heme oxygenase-1 and tissue inhibitor of metalloproteinase-4 as well as elevated peripheral neutrophil counts are associated with TB-diabetes comorbidity. *Chest, 145*, 1244–1254.

Baker, M. A., Harries, A. D., Jeon, C. Y., Hart, J. E., Kapur, A., Lonnroth, K., Ottmani, S. E., Goonesekera, S. D., & Murray, M. B. (2011). The impact of diabetes on tuberculosis treatment outcomes: A systematic review. *BMC Medicine, 9*, 81.

Baker, M. A., Lin, H. H., Chang, H. Y., & Murray, M. B. (2012). The risk of tuberculosis disease among persons with diabetes mellitus: A prospective cohort study. *Clinical Infectious Diseases, 54*, 818–825.

Bashar, M., Alcabes, P., Rom, W. N., & Condos, R. (2001). Increased incidence of multidrug-resistant tuberculosis in diabetic patients on the Bellevue Chest Service, 1987 to 1997. *Chest, 120*, 1514–1519.

Behr, M. A., Warren, S. A., Salamon, H., Hopewell, P. C., Ponce de, L. A., Daley, C. L., & Small, P. M. (1999). Transmission of Mycobacterium tuberculosis from patients smear-negative for acid-fast bacilli. *Lancet, 353*, 444–449.

Boillat-Blanco, N., Ramaiya, K. L., Mganga, M., Minja, L. T., Bovet, P., Schindler, C., Von Eckardstein, A., Gagneux, S., Daubenberger, C., Reither, K., et al. (2016). Transient hyperglycemia in patients with tuberculosis in Tanzania: Implications for diabetes screening algorithms. *The Journal of Infectious Diseases, 213*, 1163–1172.

Boucot, K. R., Dillon, E. S., Cooper, D. A., Meier, P., & Richardson, R. (1952). Tuberculosis among diabetics: The Philadelphia survey. *American Review of Tuberculosis, 65*, 1–50.

Brownlee, M. (2001). Biochemistry and molecular cell biology of diabetic complications. *Nature, 414*, 813–820.

Cheekatla, S. S., Tripathi, D., Venkatasubramanian, S., Nathella, P. K., Paidipally, P., Ishibashi, M., Welch, E., Tvinnereim, A. R., Ikebe, M., Valluri, V. L., et al. (2016). NK-CD11c+ cell crosstalk in diabetes enhances IL-6-mediated inflammation during Mycobacterium tuberculosis infection. *PLoS Pathogens, 12*, e1005972.

Dalmas, E., & Donath, M. Y. (2014). A role for interleukin-22 in the alleviation of metabolic syndrome. *Nature Medicine, 20*, 1379–1381.

Delgado-Sanchez, G., Garcia-Garcia, L., Castellanos-Joya, M., Cruz-Hervert, P., Ferreyra-Reyes, L., Ferreira-Guerrero, E., Hernandez, A., Ortega-Baeza, V. M., Montero-Campos, R., Sulca, J. A., et al. (2015). Association of pulmonary tuberculosis and diabetes in Mexico: Analysis of the national tuberculosis registry 2000-2012. *PLoS One, 10*, e0129312.

Faurholt-Jepsen, D., Aabye, M. G., Jensen, A. V., Range, N., PrayGod, G., Jeremiah, K., Changalucha, J., Faurholt-Jepsen, M., Jensen, L., Jensen, S. M., et al. (2014). Diabetes is associated with lower tuberculosis antigen-specific interferon gamma release in Tanzanian tuberculosis patients and non-tuberculosis controls. *Scandinavian Journal of Infectious Diseases, 46*, 384–391.

Fernandez-Real, J. M., & Pickup, J. C. (2012). Innate immunity, insulin resistance and type 2 diabetes. *Diabetologia, 55*, 273–278.

Fisher-Hoch, S. P., Whitney, E., McCormick, J. B., Crespo, G., Smith, B., Rahbar, M. H., & Restrepo, B. I. (2008). Type 2 diabetes and multidrug-resistant tuberculosis. *Scandinavian Journal of Infectious Diseases, 40*, 888–893.

Getahun, H., Gunneberg, C., Granich, R., & Nunn, P. (2010). HIV infection-associated tuberculosis: The epidemiology and the response. *Clinical Infectious Diseases, 50*(Suppl 3), S201–S207.

Giacco, F., & Brownlee, M. (2010). Oxidative stress and diabetic complications. *Circulation Research, 107*, 1058–1070.

Goetze, A. M., Liu, Y. D., Arroll, T., Chu, L., & Flynn, G. C. (2012). Rates and impact of human antibody glycation in vivo. *Glycobiology, 22*, 221–234.

Goldhaber-Fiebert, J. D., Jeon, C. Y., Cohen, T., & Murray, M. B. (2011). Diabetes mellitus and tuberculosis in countries with high tuberculosis burdens: Individual risks and social determinants. *International Journal of Epidemiology, 40*, 417–428.

Gomez, D. I., Twahirwa, M., Schlesinger, L. S., & Restrepo, B. I. (2013). Reduced Mycobacterium tuberculosis association with monocytes from diabetes patients that have poor glucose control. *Tuberculosis, 93*, 192–197.

Gomez-Gomez, A., Magana-Aquino, M., Lopez-Meza, S., Aranda-Alvarez, M., Diaz-Ornelas, D. E., Hernandez-Segura, M. G., Salazar-Lezama, M. A., Castellanos-Joya, M., & Noyola, D. E. (2015). Diabetes and other risk factors for multi-drug resistant tuberculosis in a Mexican population with pulmonary tuberculosis: Case control study. *Archives of Medical Research, 46*, 142–148.

Gonzalez-Curiel, I., Castaneda-Delgado, J., Lopez-Lopez, N., Araujo, Z., Hernandez-Pando, R., Gandara-Jasso, B., ias-Segura, N., Enciso-Moreno, A., & Rivas-Santiago, B. (2011). Differential expression of antimicrobial peptides in active and latent tuberculosis and its relationship with diabetes mellitus. *Human Immunology, 72*, 656–662.

Guirado, E., Schlesinger, L. S., & Kaplan, G. (2013). Macrophages in tuberculosis: Friend or foe. *Seminars in Immunopathology, 35*, 563–583.

Harris, J., & Keane, J. (2010). How tumour necrosis factor blockers interfere with tuberculosis immunity. *Clinical and Experimental Immunology, 161*, 1–9.

Hasnain, S. Z., Borg, D. J., Harcourt, B. E., Tong, H., Sheng, Y. H., Ng, C. P., Das, I., Wang, R., Chen, A. C., Loudovaris, T., et al. (2014). Glycemic control in diabetes is restored by therapeutic manipulation of cytokines that regulate beta cell stress. *Nature Medicine, 20*, 1417–1426.

Herrera, M. T., Gonzalez, Y., Hernandez-Sanchez, F., Fabian-San Miguel, G., & Torres, M. (2017). Low serum vitamin D levels in type 2 diabetes patients are associated with decreased mycobacterial activity. *BMC Infectious Diseases, 17*, 610.

Hsu, A. H., Lee, J. J., Chiang, C. Y., Li, Y. H., Chen, L. K., & Lin, C. B. (2013). Diabetes is associated with drug- resistant tuberculosis in Eastern Taiwan. *The International Journal of Tuberculosis and Lung Disease, 17*, 354–356.

Hu, F. (2011). Globalization of diabetes: The role of diet, lifestyle, and genes. *Diabetes Care, 34*, 1249–1257.

Huangfu, P., Pearson, F., Ugarte-Gil, C., & Critchley, J. (2017). Diabetes and poor tuberculosis treatment outcomes: Issues and implications in data interpretation and analysis. *The International Journal of Tuberculosis and Lung Disease, 21*, 1214–1219.

International-Diabetes-Federation. (2015). *IDF diabetes atlas* (7th ed.). Brussels, Belgium: International Diabetes Federation.

Islamoglu, H., Cao, R., Teskey, G., Gyurjian, K., Lucar, S., Fraix, M. P., Sathananthan, A., Chan, J. K., & Venketaraman, V. (2018). Effects of ReadiSorb L-GSH in altering granulomatous responses against Mycobacterium tuberculosis infection. *Journal of Clinical Medicine, 7*, pii: E40.

Jeon, C. Y., & Murray, M. B. (2008). Diabetes mellitus increases the risk of active tuberculosis: A systematic review of 13 observational studies. *PLoS Medicine, 5*, 1091–1101.

Jeon, C. Y., Murray, M. B., & Baker, M. A. (2012). Managing tuberculosis in patients with diabetes mellitus: Why we care and what we know. *Expert Review of Anti-Infective Therapy, 10*,
863–868.

Jimenez-Corona, M. E., Cruz-Hervert, L. P., Garcia-Garcia, L., Ferreyra-Reyes, L., Delgado-
Sanchez, G., Bobadilla-del-Valle, M., Canizales-Quintero, S., Ferreira-Guerrero, E., Baez-
Saldana, R., Tellez-Vazquez, N., et al. (2013). Association of diabetes and tuberculosis: Impact
on treatment and post-treatment outcomes. *Thorax, 68*, 214–220.

Jorgensen, M. E., & Faurholt-Jepsen, D. (2014). Is there an effect of glucose lowering treatment
on incidence and prognosis of tuberculosis? A systematic review. *Current Diabetes Reports,
14*, 505.

Kornfeld, H., West, K., Kane, K., Kumpatla, S., Zacharias, R. R., Martinez-Balzano, C., Li, W.,
& Viswanathan, V. (2016). High prevalence and heterogeneity of diabetes in patients with TB
in South India: A report from the effects of diabetes on tuberculosis severity (EDOTS) study.
Chest, 149, 1501–1508.

Kumar, N. P., Sridhar, R., Banurekha, V. V., Jawahar, M. S., Fay, M. P., Nutman, T. B., & Babu,
S. (2013a). Type 2 diabetes mellitus coincident with pulmonary tuberculosis is associated
with heightened systemic type 1, type 17, and other proinflammatory cytokines. *Annals of the
American Thoracic Society, 10*, 441–449.

Kumar, N. P., Sridhar, R., Banurekha, V. V., Jawahar, M. S., Nutman, T. B., & Babu, S. (2013b).
Expansion of pathogen-specific T-helper 1 and T-helper 17 cells in pulmonary tuberculosis
with coincident type 2 diabetes mellitus. *The Journal of Infectious Diseases, 208*, 739–748.

Kumar, N. P., George, P. J., Kumaran, P., Dolla, C. K., Nutman, T. B., & Babu, S. (2014).
Diminished systemic and antigen-specific type 1, type 17, and other proinflammatory cyto-
kines in diabetic and prediabetic individuals with latent Mycobacterium tuberculosis infection.
The Journal of Infectious Diseases, 210, 1670–1678.

Kumar, N. P., Banurekha, V. V., Nair, D., Kumaran, P., Dolla, C. K., & Babu, S. (2015a). Type 2
diabetes – tuberculosis co-morbidity is associated with diminished circulating levels of IL-20
subfamily of cytokines. *Tuberculosis (Edinburgh, Scotland), 95*, 707–712.

Kumar, N. P., Sridhar, R., Nair, D., Banurekha, V. V., Nutman, T. B., & Babu, S. (2015b). Type 2
diabetes mellitus is associated with altered CD8(+) T and natural killer cell function in pulmonary tuberculosis. *Immunology, 144*, 677–686.

Kumar, N. P., Moideen, K., George, P. J., Dolla, C., Kumaran, P., & Babu, S. (2016a). Coincident
diabetes mellitus modulates Th1-, Th2-, and Th17-cell responses in latent tuberculosis in an
IL-10- and TGF-beta- dependent manner. *European Journal of Immunology, 46*, 390–399.

Kumar, N. P., Moideen, K., George, P. J., Dolla, C., Kumaran, P., & Babu, S. (2016b). Impaired
cytokine but enhanced cytotoxic marker expression in Mycobacterium tuberculosis-induced
CD8+ T cells in individuals with type 2 diabetes and latent Mycobacterium tuberculosis infection. *The Journal of Infectious Diseases, 213*, 866–870.

Kumar, N. P., Moideen, K., Sivakumar, S., Menon, P. A., Viswanathan, V., Kornfeld, H., & Babu,
S. (2017a). Tuberculosis-diabetes co-morbidity is characterized by heightened systemic levels
of circulating angiogenic factors. *The Journal of Infection, 74*, 10–21.

Kumar, N. P., Moideen, K., Viswanathan, V., Sivakumar, S., Menon, P. A., Kornfeld, H., & Babu,
S. (2017b). Heightened circulating levels of antimicrobial peptides in tuberculosis-diabetes comorbidity and reversal upon treatment. *PLoS One, 12*, e0184753.

Kuo, M. C., Lin, S. H., Lin, C. H., Mao, I. C., Chang, S. J., & Hsieh, M. C. (2013). Type 2 diabetes:
An independent risk factor for tuberculosis: A nationwide population-based study. *PLoS One,
8*, e78924.

Lagman, M., Ly, J., Saing, T., Kaur Singh, M., Vera Tudela, E., Morris, D., Chi, P. T., Ochoa, C.,
Sathananthan, A., & Venketaraman, V. (2015). Investigating the causes for decreased levels of
glutathione in individuals with type II diabetes. *PLoS One, 10*, e0118436.

Lai, C. C., Lee, M. T., Lee, S. H., Hsu, W. T., Chang, S. S., Chen, S. C., & Lee, C. C. (2016). Statin
treatment is associated with a decreased risk of active tuberculosis: An analysis of a nationally
representative cohort. *Thorax, 71*, 646–651.

Leeds, I. L., Magee, M. J., Kurbatova, E. V., del, R. C., Blumberg, H. M., Leonard, M. K., & Kraft, C. S. (2012). Site of extrapulmonary tuberculosis is associated with HIV infection. *Clinical Infectious Diseases, 55*, 75–81.

Leung, C. C., Lam, T. H., Chan, W. M., Yew, W. W., Ho, K. S., Leung, G. M., Law, W. S., Tam, C. M., Chan, C. K., & Chang, K. C. (2008). Diabetic control and risk of tuberculosis: A cohort study. *American Journal of Epidemiology, 167*, 1486–1494.

Lonnroth, K., Jaramillo, E., Williams, B. G., Dye, C., & Raviglione, M. (2009). Drivers of tuberculosis epidemics: The role of risk factors and social determinants. *Social Science & Medicine, 68*, 2240–2246.

Lonnroth, K., Roglic, G., & Harries, A. D. (2014). Improving tuberculosis prevention and care through addressing the global diabetes epidemic: From evidence to policy and practice. *The Lancet Diabetes and Endocrinology, 2*, 730–739.

Lopez-Lopez, N., Martinez, A. G. R., Garcia-Hernandez, M. H., Hernandez-Pando, R., Castaneda-Delgado, J. E., Lugo-Villarino, G., Cougoule, C., Neyrolles, O., Rivas-Santiago, B., Valtierra-Alvarado, M. A., et al. (2018). Type-2 diabetes alters the basal phenotype of human macrophages and diminishes their capacity to respond, internalise, and control Mycobacterium tuberculosis. *Memórias do Instituto Oswaldo Cruz, 113*, e170326.

Magee, M. J., Bloss, E., Shin, S. S., Contreras, C., Huaman, H. A., Ticona, J. C., Bayona, J., Bonilla, C., Yagui, M., Jave, O., et al. (2013). Clinical characteristics, drug resistance, and treatment outcomes among tuberculosis patients with diabetes in Peru. *International Journal of Infectious Diseases, 17*, e404–e412.

Magee, M. J., Kempker, R. R., Kipiani, M., Gandhi, N. R., Darchia, L., Tukvadze, N., Howards, P. P., Narayan, K. M., & Blumberg, H. M. (2015). Diabetes mellitus is associated with cavities, smear grade, and multidrug- resistant tuberculosis in Georgia. *The International Journal of Tuberculosis and Lung Disease, 19*, 685–692.

Martens, G. W., Arikan, M. C., Lee, J., Ren, F., Greiner, D., & Kornfeld, H. (2007). Tuberculosis susceptibility of diabetic mice. *American Journal of Respiratory Cell and Molecular Biology, 37*, 518–524.

Martinez, N., & Kornfeld, H. (2014). Diabetes and immunity to tuberculosis. *European Journal of Immunology, 44*, 617–626.

Martinez, N., Ketheesan, N., West, K., Vallerskog, T., & Kornfeld, H. (2016). Impaired recognition of Mycobacterium tuberculosis by alveolar macrophages from diabetic mice. *The Journal of Infectious Diseases, 214*, 1629–1637.

Morton, R. (1694). *Phthisiologia, or A treatise of consumptions*. London, UK.

Muller, L. M., Gorter, K. J., Hak, E., Goudzwaard, W. L., Schellevis, F. G., Hoepelman, A. I., & Rutten, G. E. (2005). Increased risk of common infections in patients with type 1 and type 2 diabetes mellitus. *Clinical Infectious Diseases, 41*, 281–288.

Odone, A., Houben, R. M., White, R. G., & Lonnroth, K. (2014). The effect of diabetes and undernutrition trends on reaching 2035 global tuberculosis targets. *The Lancet Diabetes and Endocrinology, 2*, 754–764.

Ottmani, S. E., Murray, M. B., Jeon, C. Y., Baker, M. A., Kapur, A., Lonnroth, K., & Harries, A. D. (2010). Consultation meeting on tuberculosis and diabetes mellitus: Meeting summary and recommendations. *The International Journal of Tuberculosis and Lung Disease, 14*, 1513–1517.

Pan, S. C., Ku, C. C., Kao, D., Ezzati, M., Fang, C. T., & Lin, H. H. (2015). Effect of diabetes on tuberculosis control in 13 countries with high tuberculosis: A modelling study. *The Lancet Diabetes and Endocrinology, 3*, 323–330.

Parihar, S. P., Guler, R., Khutlang, R., Lang, D. M., Hurdayal, R., Mhlanga, M. M., Suzuki, H., Marais, A. D., & Brombacher, F. (2014). Statin therapy reduces the mycobacterium tuberculosis burden in human macrophages and in mice by enhancing autophagy and phagosome maturation. *The Journal of Infectious Diseases, 209*, 754–763.

Perez-Navarro, L. M., Fuentes-Dominguez, F. J., & Zenteno-Cuevas, R. (2015). Type 2 diabetes mellitus and its influence in the development of multidrug resistance tuberculosis in patients from southeastern Mexico. *Journal of Diabetes and its Complications, 29*, 77–82.

Perez-Navarro, L. M., Restrepo, B. I., Fuentes-Dominguez, F. J., Duggirala, R., Morales-Romero, J., Lopez-Alvarenga, J. C., Comas, I., & Zenteno-Cuevas, R. (2017). The effect size of type 2 diabetes mellitus on tuberculosis drug resistance and adverse treatment outcomes. *Tuberculosis (Edinburgh, Scotland), 103*, 83–91.

Pickup, J. C. (2004). Inflammation and activated innate immunity in the pathogenesis of type 2 diabetes. *Diabetes Care, 27*, 813–823.

Podell, B. K., Ackart, D. F., Obregon-Henao, A., Eck, S. P., Henao-Tamayo, M., Richardson, M., Orme, I. M., Ordway, D. J., & Basaraba, R. J. (2014). Increased severity of tuberculosis in Guinea pigs with type 2 diabetes: a model of diabetes-tuberculosis comorbidity. *American Journal of Pathology, 184*, 1104–1118.

Ponce-De-Leon, A., Garcia-Garcia, M. D. L., Garcia-Sancho, M. C., Gomez-Perez, F. J., Valdespino-Gomez, J. L., Olaiz-Fernandez, G., Rojas, R., Ferreyra-Reyes, L., Cano-Arellano, B., Bobadilla, M., et al. (2004). Tuberculosis and diabetes in southern Mexico. *Diabetes Care, 27*, 1584–1590.

Prada-Medina, C. A., Fukutani, K. F., Pavan Kumar, N., Gil-Santana, L., Babu, S., Lichtenstein, F., West, K., Sivakumar, S., Menon, P. A., Viswanathan, V., et al. (2017). Systems immunology of diabetes-tuberculosis comorbidity reveals signatures of disease complications. *Scientific Reports, 7*, 1999.

Reed, G. W., Choi, H., Lee, S. Y., Lee, M., Kim, Y., Park, H., Lee, J., Zhan, X., Kang, H., Hwang, S., et al. (2013). Impact of diabetes and smoking on mortality in tuberculosis. *PLoS One, 8*, e58044.

Reis-Santos, B., Locatelli, R., Horta, B. L., Faerstein, E., Sanchez, M. N., Riley, L. W., & Maciel, E. L. (2013). Socio-demographic and clinical differences in subjects with tuberculosis with and without diabetes mellitus in Brazil – a multivariate analysis. *PLoS One, 8*, e62604.

Restrepo, B. I. (2007). Convergence of the tuberculosis and diabetes epidemics: Renewal of old acquaintances. *Clinical Infectious Diseases, 45*, 436–438.

Restrepo, B. I. (2016). Metformin: Candidate host-directed therapy for tuberculosis in diabetes and non-diabetes patients. *Tuberculosis, 101*, S69–S72.

Restrepo, B. I., & Schlesinger, L. S. (2014). Impact of diabetes on the natural history of tuberculosis. *Diabetes Research and Clinical Practice, 106*, 191–199.

Restrepo, B. I., Fisher-Hoch, S. P., Crespo, J. G., Whitney, E., Perez, A., Smith, B., & McCormick, J. B. (2007). Type 2 diabetes and tuberculosis in a dynamic bi-national border population. *Epidemiology and Infection, 135*, 483–491.

Restrepo, B. I., Fisher-Hoch, S., Pino, P., Salinas, A., Rahbar, M. H., Mora, F., Cortes-Penfield, N., & McCormick, J. (2008a). Tuberculosis in poorly controlled type 2 diabetes: Altered cytokine expression in peripheral white blood cells. *Clinical Infectious Diseases, 47*, 634–641.

Restrepo, B. I., Fisher-Hoch, S., Smith, B., Jeon, S., Rahbar, M. H., & McCormick, J. (2008b). Mycobacterial clearance from sputum is delayed during the first phase of treatment in patients with diabetes. *The American Journal of Tropical Medicine and Hygiene, 79*, 541–544.

Restrepo, B. I., Camerlin, A. J., Rahbar, M. H., Wang, W., Restrepo, M. A., Zarate, I., Mora-Guzman, F., Crespo-Solis, J. G., Briggs, J., McCormick, J. B., et al. (2011). Cross-sectional assessment reveals high diabetes prevalence among newly-diagnosed tuberculosis cases. *Bulletin of the World Health Organization, 89*, 352–359.

Restrepo, B. I., Twahirwa, M., Rahbar, M. H., & Schlesinger, L. S. (2014). Phagocytosis via complement or Fc-gamma receptors is compromised in monocytes from type 2 diabetes patients with chronic hyperglycemia. *PLoS One, 9*, e92977.

Ronacher, K., Joosten, S. A., van Crevel, R., Dockrell, H. M., Walzl, G., & Ottenhoff, T. H. (2015). Acquired immunodeficiencies and tuberculosis: Focus on HIV/AIDS and diabetes mellitus. *Immunological Reviews, 264*, 121–137.

Root, H. (1934). The association of diabetes and tuberculosis. *New England Journal of Medicine, 210*, 1–13.

Russell, D. G. (2007). Who puts the tubercle in tuberculosis? *Nature Reviews. Microbiology, 5*, 39–47.

Shah, B. R., & Hux, J. E. (2003). Quantifying the risk of infectious diseases for people with diabetes. *Diabetes Care, 26*, 510–513.

Silwer, H., & Oscarsson, P. N. (1958). Incidence and coincidence of diabetes mellitus and pulmonary tuberculosis in a Swedish county. *Acta Medica Scandinavica. Supplementum, 335*, 1–48.

Singhal, A., Jie, L., Kumar, P., Hong, G. S., Leow, M. K., Paleja, B., Tsenova, L., Kurepina, N., Chen, J., Zolezzi, F., et al. (2014). Metformin as adjunct antituberculosis therapy. *Science Translational Medicine, 6*, 263ra159.

Stalenhoef, J. E., Alisjahbana, B., Nelwan, E. J., van der Ven-Jongekrijg, J., Ottenhoff, T. H., van der Meer, J. W., Nelwan, R. H., Netea, M. G., & van Crevel, R. (2008). The role of interferon-gamma in the increased tuberculosis risk in type 2 diabetes mellitus. *European Journal of Clinical Microbiology & Infectious Diseases, 27*, 97–103.

Stevenson, C. R., Critchley, J. A., Forouhi, N. G., Roglic, G., Williams, B. G., Dye, C., & Unwin, N. C. (2007a). Diabetes and the risk of tuberculosis: A neglected threat to public health? *Chronic Illness, 3*, 228–245.

Stevenson, C. R., Forouhi, N. G., Roglic, G., Williams, B. G., Lauer, J. A., Dye, C., & Unwin, N. (2007b). Diabetes and tuberculosis: The impact of the diabetes epidemic on tuberculosis incidence. *BMC Public Health, 7*, 234.

Stirban, A., Gawlowski, T., & Roden, M. (2014). Vascular effects of advanced glycation endproducts: Clinical effects and molecular mechanisms. *Molecular Metabolism, 3*, 94–108.

Su, V. Y., Su, W. J., Yen, Y. F., Pan, S. W., Chuang, P. H., Feng, J. Y., Chou, K. T., Yang, K. Y., Lee, Y. C., & Chen, T. J. (2017). Statin use is associated with a lower risk of TB. *Chest, 152*, 598–606.

Subhash, H. S., Ashwin, I., Mukundan, U., Danda, D., John, G., Cherian, A. M., & Thomas, K. (2003). Drug resistant tuberculosis in diabetes mellitus: A retrospective study from South India. *Tropical Doctor, 33*, 154–156.

Sun, Q., Zhang, Q., Xiao, H., Cui, H., & Su, B. (2012). Significance of the frequency of CD4+CD25+CD127- T-cells in patients with pulmonary tuberculosis and diabetes mellitus. *Respirology, 17*, 876–882.

Tan, K. S., Lee, K. O., Low, K. C., Gamage, A. M., Liu, Y., Tan, G. Y., Koh, H. Q., Alonso, S., & Gan, Y. H. (2012). Glutathione deficiency in type 2 diabetes impairs cytokine responses and control of intracellular bacteria. *The Journal of Clinical Investigation, 122*, 2289–2300.

The Diabetes Control and Complications Trial Research Group, Nathan, D. M., Genuth, S., Lachin, J., Cleary, P., Crofford, O., et al. (1993). The effect of intensive treatment of diabetes on the development and progression of long-term complications in insulin-dependent diabetes mellitus. *The New England Journal of Medicine, 329*, 977–986. https://doi.org/10.1056/NEJM199309303291401

Vallerskog, T., Martens, G. W., & Kornfeld, H. (2010). Diabetic mice display a delayed adaptive immune response to Mycobacterium tuberculosis. *Journal of Immunology, 184*, 6275–6282.

Viney, K., Brostrom, R., Nasa, J., Defang, R., & Kienene, T. (2014). Diabetes and tuberculosis in the Pacific Islands region. *The Lancet Diabetes and Endocrinology, 2*, 932.

Viswanathan, V., Kumpatla, S., Aravindalochanan, V., Rajan, R., Chinnasamy, C., Srinivasan, R., Selvam, J. M., & Kapur, A. (2012). Prevalence of diabetes and pre-diabetes and associated risk factors among tuberculosis patients in India. *PLoS One, 7*, e41367.

Viswanathan, V., Vigneswari, A., Selvan, K., Satyavani, K., Rajeswari, R., & Kapur, A. (2014). Effect of diabetes on treatment outcome of smear-positive pulmonary tuberculosis--a report from South India. *Journal of Diabetes and its Complications, 28*, 162–165.

Walker, C., & Unwin, N. (2010). Estimates of the impact of diabetes on the incidence of pulmonary tuberculosis in different ethnic groups in England. *Thorax, 65*, 578–581.

Walsh, M., Camerlin, A., Miles, R., Pino, P., Martinez, P., Mora-Guzman, F., Crespo-Solis, J., Fisher-Hoch, S., McCormick, J., & Restrepo, B. I. (2010). Sensitivity of interferon-gamma release assays is not compromised in tuberculosis patients with diabetes. *The International Journal of Tuberculosis and Lung Disease, 15*, 179–184.

Wang, P. D., & Lin, R. S. (2001). Drug-resistant tuberculosis in Taipei, 1996-1999. *American Journal of Infection Control, 29*, 41–47.

Wang, C. H., Yu, C. T., Lin, H. C., Liu, C. Y., & Kuo, H. P. (1999). Hypodense alveolar macrophages in patients with diabetes mellitus and active pulmonary tuberculosis. *Tubercle and Lung Disease, 79*, 235–242.

Webb, E. A., Hesseling, A. C., Schaaf, H. S., Gie, R. P., Lombard, C. J., Spitaels, A., Delport, S., Marais, B. J., Donald, K., Hindmarsh, P., et al. (2009). High prevalence of Mycobacterium tuberculosis infection and disease in children and adolescents with type 1 diabetes mellitus. *The International Journal of Tuberculosis and Lung Disease, 13*, 868–874.

Yamashiro, S., Kawakami, K., Uezu, K., Kinjo, T., Miyagi, K., Nakamura, K., & Saito, A. (2005). Lower expression of Th1-related cytokines and inducible nitric oxide synthase in mice with streptozotocin-induced diabetes mellitus infected with Mycobacterium tuberculosis. *Clinical and Experimental Immunology, 139*, 57–64.

Zhan, Y., & Jiang, L. (2015). Status of vitamin D, antimicrobial peptide cathelicidin and T helper-associated cytokines in patients with diabetes mellitus and pulmonary tuberculosis. *Experimental and Therapeutic Medicine, 9*, 11–16.

Zumla, A., Rao, M., Parida, S. K., Keshavjee, S., Cassell, G., Wallis, R., Axelsson-Robertsson, R., Doherty, M., Andersson, J., & Maeurer, M. (2015). Inflammation and tuberculosis: Host-directed therapies. *Journal of Internal Medicine, 277*, 373–387.

Recent Advances in Tuberculosis Immunodiagnostics

Imran H. Khan

Introduction

TB remains one of the world's deadliest communicable diseases with an estimated 2 billion infected with the etiologic agent *Mycobacterium tuberculosis* (*M. tb.*). In approximately 90% of the infected individuals the infection remains quiescent (or latent; LTBI), and about 10% develop active disease in their lifetime. There are approximately 10.4 million new TB cases per year, and 1.7 million die (World Health Organization 2017). A majority of the TB patients have pulmonary TB (PTB). Extrapulmonary TB (EPTB), that may affect organs other than lung (e.g., bone, skin, nervous system, urinogenital system), accounts for approximately 15–25% of all TB cases but in some regions, it may be over 40% (World Health Organization 2017; Pollett et al. 2016; Kulchavenya 2014). EPTB is often without pulmonary symptoms, and since most of the existing diagnostic tests are sputum based they are impractical for its detection. In addition to adult TB, children are highly vulnerable to infection with *M. tb.* The global burden of pediatric TB (PED-TB) was estimated to be approximately half a million or 6% of the TB burden worldwide; in high burden settings, 10–20% of all TB cases are thought to occur in children (World Health Organization 2013). National TB programs in endemic countries report low coverage of TB-care in children mainly due to the difficulty in diagnosis. Children often present with nonspecific symptoms, and diagnosis is complicated due to difficulty in obtaining sputum which is currently the main diagnostic specimen. Young children with PTB do not produce sputum, and therefore invasive methods such as nasopharyngeal or gastric aspirates are required for pulmonary TB testing; pediatric extrapulmonary TB is another major challenge. Like many other

I. H. Khan (✉)
Department of Pathology and Laboratory Medicine, School of Medicine,
University of California Davis Health System, Sacramento, CA, USA
e-mail: ihkhan@ucdavis.edu

© Springer Nature Switzerland AG 2018
V. Venketaraman (ed.), *Understanding the Host Immune Response Against Mycobacterium tuberculosis Infection*, https://doi.org/10.1007/978-3-319-97367-8_2

infectious diseases, active TB has long been known to have disproportionate occurrence in males (Guerra-Silveira and Abad-Franch 2013; Clarke et al. 1956; Frieden et al. 2000). Recent data from the endemic countries show that there may be twice as many males than females with active disease among the TB patient population (Nhamoyebonde and Leslie 2014; Rhines 2013). A variety of factors may influence this gender bias including differences in exposure to other pathogens, sex hormones and their role in modulating the response of the immune system, genetics etc. (Nhamoyebonde and Leslie 2014). It has been reported that even after factoring in a higher exposure of males, due to social conditions in the TB endemic countries that increase the likelihood of *M. tb.* transmission, the worldwide gender bias in active TB is primarily influenced by host biology (Nhamoyebonde and Leslie 2014).

Why TB is still on the rise compared to the two other major infectious diseases, AIDS and malaria: TB has surpassed AIDS in the total number of worldwide deaths (World Health Organization 2017). Among the three biggest infectious disease killers, according to the most recent count in 2016, TB caused approximately 1.7 million deaths, and AIDS and malaria caused 1.0 and 0.44 million deaths, respectively, both of which are trending down while TB deaths have been ominously on the rise (World Health Organization 2017; World Health Organization 2016). The main obstacles in eradication of TB are the following: undiagnosed disease, delayed diagnosis, limited understanding of the disease at molecular/cellular level, poor healthcare facilities, and lack of infrastructure in TB endemic countries. TB is generally curable, but in practical terms, the key problem is the current diagnostic methods such as acid-fast bacilli (AFB) microscopy and chest X-ray (CXR), and even state-of-the-art molecular tests (e.g., GeneXpert®) have been inadequate in providing capability or capacity to efficiently detect active TB patients in high disease burden countries. The resulting poor detection rates lead to mismanagement of infectious cases, further spread of infection, and possible development of drug resistance. In high burden countries, healthcare systems will substantially benefit from rapid, accurate, and cost-effective TB detection. Immune biomarker-based blood tests are promising with several advantages: (i) Blood, as opposed to sputum, provides a better testing specimen for all kinds of TB including EPTB and PED-TB, and not only adult PTB, (ii) blood tests enable rapid testing in a high-throughput format, (iii) are suitable for point-of-care testing, (iv) since *M. tb.* is not a blood-borne pathogen, blood is safer to handle than sputum (containing live, infectious *M. tb* bacilli), and (v) blood-based tests are cost-effective.

Current Diagnostics

There are a number of test types for the detection of active TB. Diagnosis of active TB in high burden countries is primarily based on sputum smear AFB microscopy and chest X-ray (CXR). When proper clinical laboratory conditions exist, the bacterial culture method is used on sputum samples. AFB microscopy has a low sensitivity

(30–70%), and specificity ranges from 93% to 98%. Due to the simplicity and ease of use, CXR is a popular choice. However, the sensitivity ranges from 67% to 77%, with specificity around 50% (Al Zahrani et al. 2000). The culture method is the gold standard for detection of *M. tb.* in patient sputum. The major drawback of the cumbersome solid culture procedures is that *M. tb.* is a slow growing organism, requiring about 4–8 weeks to obtain results; therefore, it is not used in routine TB diagnostics in clinical settings. Faster, more automated versions of the culture test in liquid media (Mycobacteria Growth Indicator Tube (MGIT) and BacT/ALERT) reduce the time-to-results to 10–14 days; however, for some samples it may still take as long as 8 weeks to obtain the final result, and it is also expensive. Culture has been estimated to confirm only 80–85% of TB cases but with a high specificity of 98% (Anonymous 2000). Because of bio-safety, contamination, and logistical issues, culture necessitates the presence of a BSL2 facility for culturing and a BSL3 for culture manipulation, that are rare in resource poor countries (World Health Organization 2007). Several molecular-based diagnostic methods for detecting *M. tb.* have been introduced over the last several years with marginal impact on worldwide TB diagnostics. Methods such as nucleic acid amplification tests (NAATs) (Safianowska et al. 2012) and loop-mediated isothermal amplification (LAMP) (Kumar et al. 2014) are also considered as rapid and accurate with improved sensitivity and specificity, but they require infrastructure and investment which is not in affordable range for endemic countries, a majority of which are resource poor. Cepheid's molecular test for TB diagnostics (Xpert MTB/RIF or GeneXpert®) was endorsed in 2010 by the WHO to be used as an initial diagnostic for those individuals suspected of having MDR-TB or HIV-associated TB (World Health Organization 2010). A key limitation is that this assay has a capacity of 20 samples per day in the typical 4 cassette configuration. This low-throughput capacity for testing the high volumes that are needed in endemic countries may result in longer wait times for the patient.

Standard of practice and its limitations: In clinical settings, in most endemic countries, the frontline TB diagnostic test is AFB microscopy which suffers from low and variable sensitivity (Fig. 1a). Culture is sparingly used because of the long wait time for results. As a consequence, the percentage of bacteriologically confirmed cases in most TB endemic countries is underwhelming, typically around 50%, while half of TB patients depend solely on clinical diagnosis (World Health Organization 2015). Clinical diagnosis in turn depends on the training and experience of the physician and quality of CXR findings suggestive of TB, both of which vary widely from country to country and clinic to clinic.

Limitations of sputum as the diagnostic specimen: Sputum has been the main focus of TB diagnostics for a long time and continues to be so for the development of new diagnostics. The first limitation is that sputum is not an appropriate diagnostic specimen for EPTB which is estimated to account for approximately 15–25% of all TB cases (likely an underestimate since EPTB is difficult to diagnose). In addition, children often have difficulty producing proper sputum sample; PEDTB accounts for 6–20% of TB. Therefore, in roughly a third of all TB cases, sputum is not a practical diagnostic specimen.

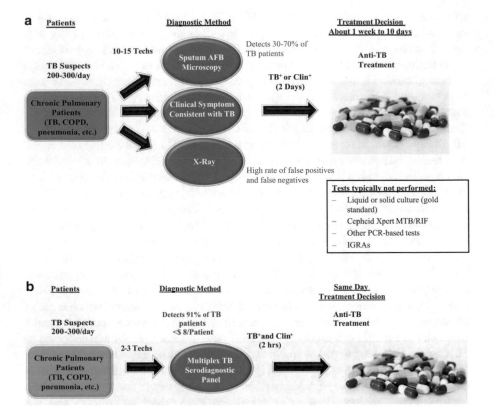

Fig. 1 (**a**) Work flow under standard of practice diagnostics in high burden countries. (**b**) Multiplex serology and proposed TB diagnostic work flow

Immune Responses in TB Patients

The outcome of *M. tb.* infection is increasingly viewed as a spectrum ranging from LTBI with no symptoms (noninfectious) to full blown active disease (infectious) (Esmail et al. 2012; Barry 3rd et al. 2009). The host immune responses play a pivotal role in determining the infection or disease status over this spectrum which broadly results in one of the following outcomes: (i) the infection may be cleared in the exposed individual, (ii) infection remains contained in well-formed lung granulomas leading to a latent state which happens in a majority of infected individuals (about 90%), (iii) breakdown of granuloma leading to progression from latency to active-disease (10% of infected) where the disease may range in severity from subclinical (with little to no symptoms) to overtly morbid (morbidity itself may range in severity from mild to extremely debilitating). The immune responses in the infected host typically remain strong even after the spectrum has shifted from latency to active disease. These immune responses are a rich source of TB immunological biomarkers (Walzl et al. 2011).

Cytokines and chemokines: TB is increasingly viewed as an imbalance of host immune responses that transition from protection against *M. tb.* infection to disease resulting in immunopathology leading to active disease (Kaufmann and Parida 2008; Dorhoi et al. 2011; Modlin and Bloom 2013). In the initial stages of infection, where *M. tb.* infects the lung, it is taken up by alveolar macrophages and dendritic cells (DCs), triggering an inflammatory response (Sasindran and Torrelles 2011; Pieters 2008). This is followed by the recruitment of monocytes and polymorphonuclear neutrophils to the site of infection; these cells express diverse antimicrobial effector molecules to activate macrophages and escalate the inflammatory process (Korbel et al. 2008). Antigen presenting DCs activate T lymphocytes in the lymph node, which then migrate to the site of infection and proliferate, leading to the formation of granulomas, a hallmark of *M. tb.* infection (Sasindran and Torrelles 2011). About 10% of infected individuals exhibit active TB, whereas the remaining *M. tb.* infected people harbor *M. tb.* in a dormant (latent) state without clinical symptoms. In a small proportion of individuals with latent infection, the bacterium may reactivate months or years later and produce disease (Kleinnijenhuis et al. 2011). In active pulmonary TB, areas of high lymphoid cell activity, arranged in tertiary lymphoid structures develop around lung granulomas and have been suggested to mimic lymphoid organs in their function (Kaufmann and Parida 2008). To define pathologic mechanisms of TB, the roles of cytokines and chemokines have been extensively studied (Kaufmann and Parida 2008; Dheda et al. 2010). Cytokines are immunomodulating agents secreted by specific cells of the immune system that mediate interactions between cells and are thus required for an integrated response to a variety of stimuli in immune and inflammatory processes (Feghali and Wright 1997). Cytokines are grouped in different classes such as interleukins, lymphokines, and cell signaling molecules. They play a role in many important biological activities, including cell proliferation, activation, death, and differentiation. In TB, cytokine/chemokine dynamics play a key role in the disease outcome (O'Garra et al. 2013). Consistent with the observation of gender bias in active TB patients, studies in other infectious diseases where more prevalent and severe disease occurred in males in comparison to females have been reported, and the bias appears to be related to differential immune responses due to the influence of sex hormones on the immune system, exerted through cytokines/chemokines (Nhamoyebonde and Leslie 2014; Marriott and Huet-Hudson 2006; Bernin and Lotter 2014). Similarly, in TB, influence of sex hormones on the immune system appears to reflect the gender bias toward males in the pathogenesis of active disease (Nhamoyebonde and Leslie 2014).

Cytokines/chemokines can be pro- or anti-inflammatory, are involved in both paracrine and autocrine pathways, and are grouped into different classes, such as interleukins, lymphokines, chemokines, and cell signaling molecules (Dinarello 2000). Proinflammatory cytokines help in the control of *M. tb.* infection, but they also play a crucial role during the chronic (latent) infection stage, dictating the pathogenesis of the disease (Flynn and Chan 2001). Tumor necrosis factor alpha

(TNF-α), interleukin-12 (IL-12), and gamma interferon (IFN-γ) are central cytokines in the regulatory and effector phases of the immune response to *M. tuberculosis (Boom* et al. 2003). Alveolar macrophages and dendritic cells release inflammatory cytokines such as TNF-α, IL-12, and IL-23 along with a variety of chemokines, including C-C motif ligand 2 (CCL2), CCL5, and C-X-C motif ligand 8 (CXCL8). The Th1 response, important for granuloma assembly, is triggered by the production of IL-12 and IL-23 by DCs (Sasindran and Torrelles 2011). Activated T cells regulate this flow of inflammatory events by secreting IFN-γ and IL-2, which activate alveolar macrophages to produce a variety of substances involved in growth inhibition and killing of mycobacteria (Cooper 2009). Immune responses to *M. tb.* infection are downregulated by the production of anti-inflammatory cytokines such as IL-4, IL-10, and transforming growth factor β (TGF-β) (Sharma and Bose 2001). In TB patients, patterns of cytokines and chemokines detected in the blood circulation can provide evidence of infection and/or disease without direct analysis of tissue from the affected organ(s) (e.g., lung biopsy). In TB patients, patterns of cytokines and chemokines detected in the blood circulation can provide evidence of infection and/or disease without direct analysis of tissue from the affected organ(s) (e.g., lung biopsy) (Yu et al. 2012; Mihret et al. 2013). It has been reported that these patterns are different in male and female patients, for example, female patients contain significantly higher levels of CXCL9 (MIG) and CXCL10 (IP-10), while males contained higher levels of PDGF-BB (Chavez et al. 2016).

Antibodies: For decades, cell-mediated immunity by T cells (involving cytokines/chemokines) and mononuclear cells had come to be known as the main host immune response in TB immunity as well as in shaping the spectrum of infection and disease. Antibodies were not considered important. This general theme was borne out in studies done in TB patients and experimentally infected animal models (e.g., mouse, guinea pig). However, in the recent years, the value of humoral immune responses in TB immunity has emerged as an important aspect of host response, based on a number of studies highlighting the role of B cells and antibodies. These studies have shown that in addition to cell-mediated immunity, humoral immunity plays a major role (Lu et al. 2016; Achkar et al. 2015). Critically, these studies have demonstrated the importance of the cooperative roles of innate, humoral, and cellular immune responses. B cells, and their influence on the TB immunity through the production of antibodies, are now considered important players in the host defenses (Lu et al. 2016; Achkar et al. 2015). In addition to production of antibodies crucial for TB immunity, B cells may also contribute to immune responses through antigen presentation and cytokine production (Achkar et al. 2015). A functional role of antibodies in TB was recently reported suggesting Fc-receptor-mediated antibody effector function; this study further demonstrated that antibody profiles in LTBI and active disease are distinct, revealing the functional role of antibodies in latency and disease (Lu et al. 2016).

Rationale for the Development of Novel Immunodiagnostic Tests

Infected individuals and TB patients mount immune responses that play an important role in latency and disease. These responses can be exploited for development of novel immunodiagnostic tools. Tuberculin skin test (TST) developed a century ago (and still actively used in many parts of the world) takes advantage of the host responses in infected individuals. However, the test suffers from sensitivity and specificity issues. Modern, more refined, in vitro versions, that have been developed to avoid measuring immune responses to BCG vaccination and nontuberculous *Mycobacteria* (NTB), are called interferon-γ release assays (IGRA). In IGRAs, blood is exposed to antigens (e.g., ESAT-6 and CFP-10) specific for *M. tb.* complex. T cells in the host blood exposed to *M. tb.* infection respond by producing IFNγ that can be measured. IGRAs have high sensitivity but do not discriminate between immune responses in LTBI and active disease (Farhat et al. 2006). Therefore, in TB endemic countries, where LTBI may be common in the general population, IGRAs are not suitable for routine TB diagnostics. Host immune responses, in addition, produce antibodies and cytokines/ chemokines that are released into the circulation, and can be assayed without stimulation of blood. In addition, detection of antibody responses against *M. tb.* antigens, carefully selected to avoid nonspecific interactions (associated with BCG vaccination, NTB infection, and LTBI elicited background immune responses), can be used for diagnostic purposes for active TB, by the use of highly sensitive and specific immunoassays. It has been demonstrated in several studies that well-defined profiles of antibodies specific to active disease, detected by the multiplex immunoassay formats, may have utility for the development of TB diagnostic tools (Khan et al. 2011; Kunnath-Velayudhan et al. 2010; Lyashchenko et al. 2007; Lyashchenko et al. 2017).

Limitations of the current antibody based Immunoassays for TB: Several antibody based serology tests have been introduced. The lack of affordable, rapid, and precise diagnostic tools and the ease of serology assays have led to the use of a large number of commercial serological tests, in the lateral flow (immunochemistry) and ELISA formats (Singh and Katoch 2011). Serology tests for active TB are based on antibody recognition of antigens of *M. tb.* There are a large number of commercially available serological tests; 60 tests in the lateral flow (immunochemistry) format and 13 in the ELISA format (Singh and Katoch 2011). The key to accurate diagnosis using serology is the correct choice of antigen(s) that are able to differentiate between active disease, latent infection, LTBI, and BCG vaccination while maintaining high sensitivity and specificity. Importantly, individual TB patients generate antibodies to different *M. tb.* antigens, and therefore, development of good serology tests requires combinations of several antigens. For this reason, a majority of the current serology based tests, which typically contain one or two antigens, suffer from low sensitivity. Furthermore, a majority of the serology tests in the market have not been extensively tested and clinically validated and are therefore unreliable for TB diagnostics (Flynn and Chan 2001; Boom et al. 2003; Cooper 2009; Sharma and Bose 2001; Yu et al. 2012; Mihret et al. 2013; Chavez et al. 2016).

Novel Antibody-Based Immunoassays

The attractiveness of serology tests is that they are simpler to perform, faster to results than sputum- based methodologies such as microscopy, culture, or PCR, and lack the infectious sputum component. However, the current commercial serology tests have poor performance with inconsistent sensitivity and specificity (Steingart et al. 2007a). For these reasons, the World Health Organization (WHO) issued a negative recommendation on existing serology tests based on a systematic evidence-based process. However, it is important to note that the negative recommendation only applies to serology tests that are currently on the market (Singh and Katoch 2011; Steingart et al. 2007a; Anonymous 2011; Dowdy et al. 2011; Steingart et al. 2009; Steingart et al. 2011; Steingart et al. 2007b). It is therefore important to develop new tests taking advantage of the advances in scientific knowledge and availability of newer technologies. TB serology tests that are based on sound scientific principles and proper clinical validation and address the limitations to overcome the sensitivity and specificity challenges of the existing ones would be useful in curtailing the spread of TB. A major challenge in the use of antibodies in TB patients for diagnostic purposes is that not all TB patients make antibodies to the same *M .tb.* antigens. The knowledge of *M. tb.* genome and the details of open-reading frames have been helpful in a systematic search for the useful antigens for the development of multiplex panels for TB serology. The complete genome sequences of *M. tb.* (H37Rv, virulent laboratory strain) have been determined (Cole et al. 1998). More recently, specific and sensitive TB diagnostic tests have been developed by taking advantage of advances in sequencing and annotation of the *M. tb.* genome which has revealed approximately 4,000 open-reading frames (http://genolist.pasteur.fr/TubercuList/).

Development of new antibody tests: A comprehensive study of the entire proteome of *M. tb.* has highlighted antigenic potential of individual proteins reacting to sera from TB patients collected from several countries around the world. This study revealed that a limited number of proteins expressed by the entire genome of *M. tb.* react to sera from TB patients, thus narrowing down the number of useful antigens to 13 (Kunnath-Velayudhan et al. 2010). These results suggest that although the traditional immune-assay formats (e.g., ELISA, Western Blot) are not practical for use in TB diagnostics since several antigens are required for high sensitivity, modern technologies that enable multiplexing can be employed for TB serology. Indeed multiplex approaches have enabled successful development of serological tests for TB on a range of technology platforms (e.g., protein chip array, lateral flow, microbead suspension array) (Khan et al. 2011; Kunnath-Velayudhan et al. 2010; Lyashchenko et al. 2007; Lyashchenko et al. 2018; Kunnath-Velayudhan and Gennaro 2011; Khan et al. 2008; Khaliq et al. 2017). Panels of multiple *M. tb.* antigens detect antibodies in TB patients to yield high sensitivity in serological testing. A variety of technology platforms (e.g., protein chip array (PCA), microbead suspension array (MSA)), have been developed and studied (Kunnath-Velayudhan et al. 2010; Khaliq et al. 2017). In these multiplex assays, the detection of antibodies to even a single antigen out of the entire panel gives a positive result for TB. It is important to note that in separate studies performed in TB patients, many of the antibody panels (antigens) were found to be common, while a few others are different (Table 1). The differences could be due to antigen presentation in each technology platform. In PCA (a two-dimensional platform), epitope presentation is likely to be different than the MSA platform where antigen-coupled microbeads are suspended in liquid and are therefore likely to be exposed to sample in all directions. Another suspension bead array platform (Cytometric Bead Array (CBA), Becton Dickinson) performed very similar to MSA (unpublished, this author). Studies in animal models are shown (Table 1) and discussed further in more detail below. Briefly, results in nonhuman primate and rabbit models displayed similarities in the antibody profiles with many antibodies in common. Importantly, profiles in the two animal models share similarities with TB patients for a number of common antibodies. Together, the results in TB patients and animal model studies suggest that humoral immune responses against *M. tb.* are similar, and the antibody profiles shown represent a majority of the important antibodies. Therefore, a panel of selected *M. tb.* antigens, that can detect specific antibodies in a majority of TB patients but not in nontuberculous respiratory diseases, could be developed and clinically validated for TB diagnostics that would be superior in sensitivity to not only the currently marketed TB serology tests but also AFP microscopy (low sensitivity), the first-line TB diagnostic test recommended by WHO.

Antibody-based immunoassays in animal models: Several experimental animal models are available for studying TB (e.g., nonhuman primates, guinea pig, mouse, rabbit, and others). The nonhuman primate model represents human TB most closely (Flynn et al. 2003; Flynn 2006). Studies on experimentally infected nonhuman primates have been performed to demonstrate the utility of antibody profiling in characterization of humoral immune responses in infection and disease (Lyashchenko et al. 2007; Khan et al. 2008). More recently, it has been demonstrated that multiplex profiles of anti-*M. tb.* antibodies are useful in the detection of active disease in natural TB outbreak as well as in experimentally infected nonhuman primates (Table 1) (Ravindran et al. 2014). In addition to the use of nonhuman primates as an animal model for TB research, TB is a serious concern in the health management of primate colonies, and animals used in research are required to be routinely tested for TB a few times a year. To that end, the above multiplex antibody detection assay has been clinically validated and commercialized through Research Animal Diagnostics, Charles River (Wilmington, MA), for TB monitoring in animal colonies (manuscript in preparation, this author). In addition, antibody profiles have been studied in the experimental rabbit model. Rabbit model of pulmonary TB also manifests various stages of disease pathology consistently, and closely, to human TB (Converse et al. 1996; Subbian 2015). Antibodies against *M. tb.* antigens, to assess their utility in characterizing the host immune responses in a rabbit model of pulmonary TB by multiplex immunoassays, have been studied; a profile of antibodies similar to those in TB patients and monkey model have been reported (Table 1) (Dehnad et al. 2016). Profiles of antibodies useful in TB diagnostics in other animal

Table 1 Diagnostically valuable antibody profiles in TB patients and animal models (nonhuman primate and rabbit)

Antibodies (antigens)	TB patients (PCA) (Kunnath-Velayudhan et al. 2010)	TB patients (MSA) (Khaliq et al. 2017)	Nonhuman primate TB outbreak (MSA) (Ravindran et al. 2014)	Nonhuman primate experimental (MSA) (Ravindran et al. 2014)	Rabbit experimental (MSA) (Dehnad et al. 2016)
Rv3881	X	X	X	X	
Rv0934	X	X	X	X	X
RV3804c	X	X	X	X	X
Rv2031c	X	X	X	X	X
Rv3874	X	X	X	X	
Rv1860	X	X			X
Rv1984c	X	X			
Rv1980c	X	X			
Rv1886c		X	X	X	X
Rv2875		X			X
Rv3841		X	X	X	
Rv1926c		X			
Rv3616c	X				
Rv1411c	X				
Rv3864	X				
Rv0632c	X				
Rv2873	X				
Rv3875			X	X	X
Rv3874–3875			X	X	X
Rv0831		X			
Rv2220		X			
Rv0054		X			
Rv1099		X			
Rv0129c		X			

MSA Microbead suspension array, *PCA* Protein chip array – two-dimensional

species, for example, elephants, cattle, and various species of deer, infected with *M. tb.* or *M. bovis*, have also been extensively studied and their utility in TB diagnostics has been demonstrated (Lyashchenko et al. 2017; Lyashchenko et al. 2018; Waters et al. 2017). Of particular value is the antibody profiling in cattle with TB, even when the animals were nonreactive to TST (Waters et al. 2017).

Cytokine/chemokine immunoassays in unstimulated blood from TB patients: Pulmonary TB is an inflammatory disease with involvement of many cytokines/chemokines (Kaufmann and Parida 2008; Dorhoi et al. 2011; Dheda et al. 2010). Direct measurement of cytokines/chemokines in patient plasma offers more practical means to study host immune responses in active TB than in stimulated blood, as in the format represented by IGRAs (Yu et al. 2012; Mihret et al. 2013). In addition, it offers an opportunity to investigate a more natural perspective on the immune responses in active disease. It has been demonstrated by multiplex analysis that amounts of ten cytokines/chemokines could be readily quantitated in plasma samples from active TB patients (Ravindran et al. 2013). Of these, a profile of nine cytokines/chemokines dominated the patient plasma consisting of IL-18, IFNγ, CXCL10, CXCL9, GCSF, IL-6, CXCL1, VEGF, and PDGFBB. An interesting observation in this study was that samples from patients with weak humoral response (low levels of antibodies against only a few *M. tb.* antigens) contained higher amounts of cytokines/chemokines in a larger proportion of patients, while patients with stronger humoral response (high levels of several antibodies) contained fewer cytokines/chemokines and in low amounts. These results suggest that among TB patients, those individuals who mount a strong humoral response contain weaker cytokine/chemokine responses and vice versa. Measurements of cytokines/chemokines could also be valuable as biomarkers to monitor efficacy of therapy in TB patients. Cytokines/chemokines are small, fragile proteins and therefore, a decrease in their amount may reflect a corresponding reduction in TB-related lung inflammation in patients responding to successful therapy (Chavez et al. 2016; Riou et al. 2012). TB treatment is drawn out (6 months) during which period it is difficult to monitor treatment efficacy and patient compliance (Munro et al. 2007). It has been shown that in blood samples taken from patients under anti-tuberculous therapy (ATT) at the time of TB diagnosis (0 month) and over several months during the treatment (2 and 4 months) several cytokines/chemokines displayed drastic reduction in majority of the successfully treated patients as early as 2 months post-treatment, despite differences in the amounts in male and female patients at the time of diagnosis; amounts decreased further at 4 months post-ATT (Chavez et al. 2016). These results suggest that clinically validated cytokine/chemokine immunoassays could be useful in the clinical follow-up of patients on ATT, to monitor treatment success at early time points. An early identification of treatment failure may indicate patient noncompliance to ATT or suggest multidrug resistance (MDR).

Future Directions for Blood-Based TB Diagnostics

There is an urgent need for the development of new diagnostic tests that are not only sensitive and specific but also deliver a diagnostic capacity required in TB endemic countries, particularly in those with high disease burden. It is important to note that many other nontuberculous respiratory diseases (e.g., chronic obstructive pulmonary disease (COPD), chronic bronchitis, lung cancer) have clinical presentation similar to TB and patients suffering from these diseases are generally considered to be TB suspects. In clinical settings in endemic countries, approximately 10–20% of TB suspects get diagnosed with TB. Therefore, to find 10 million new TB cases worldwide every year, 50–100 million TB suspects need to be tested. To deal with such staggering numbers of patients, high-throughput testing systems are needed. Because

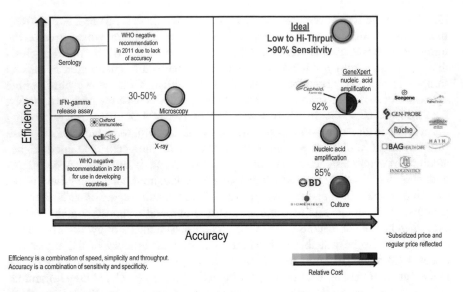

Fig. 2 Tuberculosis diagnostics landscape

majority of TB patients live in the 22 high-burden countries, most of which are resource poor, the new diagnostic tests must also be cost-effective. The current landscape of TB diagnostic tests is shown in Fig. 2. Sputum culture is the gold standard and all other diagnostic tests are benchmarked against it. The difficulty is that the gold standard itself is about 85% sensitive (Anonymous 2000). This means that a diagnostic test benchmarked only against culture and determined to have 100% sensitivity is likely not to be more than 85% sensitive. An additional difficulty is that because approximately 15–25% of TB is EPTB and 6–20% is PEDTB, broadly a third of the world's TB cannot be detected by sputum-based tests. These limitations add up and using sputum-based tests may result in missing about 40–50% of all TB cases. Under these considerations, it is hard to avoid the conclusion that the most accurate of sputum-based tests may not detect much more than 50–60% of all TB cases.

Blood-based tests use a sample specimen that represents systemic circulation, whereas sputum specimen represents only the pulmonary component. In addition, blood-based immunodiagnostic approach can deliver high-throughput tests with adequate capacity, at a low cost. However, TB serology tests are not free of controversy. This is largely due to the low sensitivity and specificity problems of the existing tests that are not rigorously validated. As discussed in detail above, several studies have demonstrated that multiplex serology is a promising option where a panel of selected *M. tb.* antigens can be used to detect antibodies in serum or plasma of patients such that if a sample contained antibodies against one of the validated antigens, the patient would be positive for active TB. In this regard, a field study using 11 *M. tb.* antigens, selected for the detection of active TB, performed in two endemic countries, India (ranked first with 27% of world's TB – 2.8 million new cases per year) and Pakistan (ranked fifth worldwide), has demonstrated high sensitivity (91% overall sensitivity) (95% and 88% sensitivity in AFB microscopy positive and negative TB patients, respectively) and specificity (96% specific in COPD patients) (Khaliq et al. 2017). Similar overall antibody profiles with similar results were obtained in a separate study performed in Uganda (Shete et al. 2017). Importantly, in the multiplex serology study performed in Pakistan which included microbiologically unconfirmed TB patients (negative by sputum-based AFB microscopy and culture), this test demonstrated 87% sensitivity. For the clinical diagnosis of these TB patients, the subjects were monitored for response to ATT in follow-up clinical examinations, and at the conclusion of 6 months of Directly Observed Treatment Short-Course (DOTS) when they were declared cured of TB (Khaliq et al. 2017). It is critical that more studies be performed where microbiologically (sputum based) unconfirmed, clinically diagnosed TB patients are included in the trials. A summary of results and comparison of the multiplex serology test that included microbiologically unconfirmed but clinically diagnosed TB patients, with other leading TB diagnostic tests, are shown in Table 2. Based on these results, a clinical validation trial for all forms of TB (PTB, EPTB, and PEDTB) has been initiated in India after approval of the study plan by the Indian Council for Medical Research (ICMR, Delhi). Under the guidance of ICMR, the trial is being performed at three different sites in India and is expected to be concluded in 2019. Upon clinical validation and the final approval, the multiplex serology test would be posi-

Table 2 Comparison of sensitivity and specificity of multiplex TB serodiagnostic panel containing 11 antigens to established sputum-based tests

	Multiplex TB serodiagnostic panel (11 antigens)	Sputum smear microscopy	Culture	Cepheid Xpert MTB/RIF (Boehme et al. 2010)
AFB[+,a] culture[+] sensitivity	95%	100%	–	98%
AFB,[-] culture[+] sensitivity	88%	0%	100%	72%
AFB,[-] culture[-] sensitivity	87%	0%	0%	0%
Sensitivity (overall)	91%	30–70%	100% (85%)	92%
Specificity	96%	93–99%	98%	99%
Time to results	2 h	2 days	2–8 weeks	2 h
Patient throughput/day	360[b]	20 slides/tech[c]	–	20
Patient sample source	Blood	Sputum	Sputum	Sputum
Approx. price (US$)	$5–7	$5–10	$20–40	$10/$28–86[d]

[a]AFB = Acid-fast bacilli sputum smear microscopy; AFB[+] denotes positive result and AFB[-] denotes negative result
[b]Throughput based on single instrument in 8 h day
[c]WHO recommended maximum slides to be viewed by a single technician per day
[d]Subsidized price (public sector) and regular price (private sector) reflected (Puri et al. 2016)

tioned to improve the clinical work flow at hospitals and diagnostic laboratories in India (Fig. 1b). This multiplex serology test can be performed with scalability from 1 to 360 patients per day and is amenable to automation for higher (1000s per day) throughput, thus enabling a scalable clinical work flow model for TB endemic countries. Additionally, this test is adaptable to a point-of-care multiplex serology platform that could be used in a small laboratory or a doctor's office. Taken together, the above discussion suggests that well-defined antibody profiles in blood, analyzed by an appropriate technology platform and validated in clinical trials, offer a valuable approach to TB diagnostics in endemic countries. The application of this multiplex system, in high-throughput or point-of-care format, for blood-based TB testing, is cost effective with an estimated commercial price of under US$8 to the end-user.

References

Achkar, J. M., Chan, J., & Casadevall, A. (2015). B cells and antibodies in the defense against Mycobacterium tuberculosis infection. *Immunological Reviews, 264*, 167–181.

Al Zahrani, K., Al Jahdali, H., Poirier, L., Rene, P., Gennaro, M. L., & Menzies, D. (2000). Accuracy and utility of commercially available amplification and serologic tests for the diagnosis of minimal pulmonary tuberculosis. *American Journal of Respiratory and Critical Care Medicine, 162*, 1323–1329.

Anonymous. (2000). Diagnostics standards and classification of tuberculosis in adults and children. This official statement of the American Thoracic Society and The Centers of Disease Control and Prevention was adopted by the ATS Board of Directors, July 1999. This statement was endorsed by the Infectious Disease Society of America, September 1999. *American Journal of Respiratory and Critical Care Medicine, 161*, 1376–1395.

Anonymous. (2011). *Commercial serodiagnostic tests for diagnosis of tuberculosis: Policy statement.* Geneva: World Health Organization.

Barry, C. E., 3rd, Boshoff, H. I., Dartois, V., Dick, T., Ehrt, S., Flynn, J., Schnappinger, D., Wilkinson, R. J., & Young, D. (2009). The spectrum of latent tuberculosis: Rethinking the biology and intervention strategies. *Nature Reviews. Microbiology, 7*, 845–855.

Bernin, H., & Lotter, H. (2014). Sex bias in the outcome of human tropical infectious diseases: Influence of steroid hormones. *The Journal of Infectious Diseases, 209*(Suppl 3), S107–S113.

Boehme, C. C., Nabeta, P., Hillemann, D., Nicol, M. P., Shenai, S., Krapp, F., Allen, J., Tahirli, R., Blakemore, R., Rustomjee, R., Milovic, A., Jones, M., O'Brien, S. M., Persing, D. H., Ruesch-Gerdes, S., Gotuzzo, E., Rodrigues, C., Alland, D., & Perkins, M. D. (2010). Rapid molecular detection of tuberculosis and rifampin resistance. *The New England Journal of Medicine, 363*, 1005–1015.

Boom, W. H., Canaday, D. H., Fulton, S. A., Gehring, A. J., Rojas, R. E., & Torres, M. (2003). Human immunity to M. tuberculosis: T cell subsets and antigen processing. *Tuberculosis (Edinburgh, Scotland), 83*, 98–106.

Chavez, K., Ravindran, R., Dehnad, A., & Khan, I. H. (2016). Gender biased immune-biomarkers in active tuberculosis and correlation of their profiles to efficacy of therapy. *Tuberculosis (Edinburgh, Scotland), 99*, 17–24.

Clarke, W. G., Cochrane, A. L., & Miall, W. E. (1956). Results of a chest x-ray survey in the Vale of Glamorgan; a study of an agricultural community. *Tubercle, 37*, 417–425.

Cole, S. T., Brosch, R., Parkhill, J., Garnier, T., Churcher, C., Harris, D., Gordon, S. V., Eiglmeier, K., Gas, S., Barry, C. E., 3rd, Tekaia, F., Badcock, K., Basham, D., Brown, D., Chillingworth, T., Connor, R., Davies, R., Devlin, K., Feltwell, T., Gentles, S., Hamlin, N., Holroyd, S.,

Hornsby, T., Jagels, K., Krogh, A., McLean, J., Moule, S., Murphy, L., Oliver, K., Osborne, J., Quail, M. A., Rajandream, M. A., Rogers, J., Rutter, S., Seeger, K., Skelton, J., Squares, R., Squares, S., Sulston, J. E., Taylor, K., Whitehead, S., & Barrell, B. G. (1998). Deciphering the biology of Mycobacterium tuberculosis from the complete genome sequence. *Nature, 393*, 537–544.

Converse, P. J., Dannenberg, A. M., Jr., Estep, J. E., Sugisaki, K., Abe, Y., Schofield, B. H., & Pitt, M. L. (1996). Cavitary tuberculosis produced in rabbits by aerosolized virulent tubercle bacilli. *Infection and Immunity, 64*, 4776–4787.

Cooper, A. M. (2009). Cell-mediated immune responses in tuberculosis. *Annual Review of Immunology, 27*, 393–422.

Dehnad, A., Ravindran, R., Subbian, S., & Khan, I. H. (2016). Development of immune-biomarkers of pulmonary tuberculosis in a rabbit model. *Tuberculosis (Edinburgh, Scotland), 101*, 1–7.

Dheda, K., Schwander, S. K., Zhu, B., van Zyl-Smit, R. N., & Zhang, Y. (2010). The immunology of tuberculosis: From bench to bedside. *Respirology, 15*, 433–450.

Dinarello, C. A. (2000). Proinflammatory cytokines. *Chest, 118*, 503–508.

Dorhoi, A., Reece, S. T., & Kaufmann, S. H. (2011). For better or for worse: The immune response against Mycobacterium tuberculosis balances pathology and protection. *Immunological Reviews, 240*, 235–251.

Dowdy, D. W., Steingart, K. R., & Pai, M. (2011). Serological testing versus other strategies for diagnosis of active tuberculosis in India: A cost-effectiveness analysis. *PLoS Medicine, 8*, e1001074.

Esmail, H., Barry, C. E., 3rd, & Wilkinson, R. J. (2012). Understanding latent tuberculosis: The key to improved diagnostic and novel treatment strategies. *Drug Discovery Today, 17*, 514–521.

Farhat, M., Greenaway, C., Pai, M., & Menzies, D. (2006). False-positive tuberculin skin tests: What is the absolute effect of BCG and non-tuberculous mycobacteria? *The International Journal of Tuberculosis and Lung Disease, 10*, 1192–1204.

Feghali, C. A., & Wright, T. M. (1997). Cytokines in acute and chronic inflammation. *Frontiers in Bioscience, 2*, d12–d26.

Flynn, J. L. (2006). Lessons from experimental Mycobacterium tuberculosis infections. *Microbes and Infection, 8*, 1179–1188.

Flynn, J. L., & Chan, J. (2001). Immunology of tuberculosis. *Annual Review of Immunology, 19*, 93–129.

Flynn, J. L., Capuano, S. V., Croix, D., Pawar, S., Myers, A., Zinovik, A., & Klein, E. (2003). Non-human primates: A model for tuberculosis research. *Tuberculosis (Edinburgh, Scotland), 83*, 116–118.

Frieden, T. R., Lerner, B. H., & Rutherford, B. R. (2000). Lessons from the 1800s: Tuberculosis control in the new millennium. *Lancet, 355*, 1088–1092.

Guerra-Silveira, F., & Abad-Franch, F. (2013). Sex bias in infectious disease epidemiology: Patterns and processes. *PLoS One, 8*, e62390.

Kaufmann, S. H., & Parida, S. K. (2008). Tuberculosis in Africa: Learning from pathogenesis for biomarker identification. *Cell Host & Microbe, 4*, 219–228.

Khaliq, A., Ravindran, R., Hussainy, S. F., Krishnan, V. V., Ambreen, A., Yusuf, N. W., Irum, S., Rashid, A., Jamil, M., Zaffar, F., Chaudhry, M. N., Gupta, P. K., Akhtar, M. W., & Khan, I. H. (2017). Field evaluation of a blood based test for active tuberculosis in endemic settings. *PLoS One, 12*, e0173359.

Khan, I. H., Ravindran, R., Yee, J., Ziman, M., Lewinsohn, D. M., Gennaro, M. L., Flynn, J. L., Goulding, C. W., DeRiemer, K., Lerche, N. W., & Luciw, P. A. (2008). Profiling antibodies to Mycobacterium tuberculosis by multiplex microbead suspension arrays for serodiagnosis of tuberculosis. *Clinical and Vaccine Immunology, 15*, 433–438.

Khan, I. H., Ravindran, R., Krishnan, V. V., Awan, I. N., Rizvi, S. K., Saqib, M. A., Shahzad, M. I., Tahseen, S., Ireton, G., Goulding, C. W., Felgner, P., DeRiemer, K., Khanum, A., & Luciw, P. A. (2011). Plasma antibody profiles as diagnostic biomarkers for tuberculosis. *Clinical and Vaccine Immunology, 18*, 2148–2153.

Kleinnijenhuis, J., Oosting, M., Joosten, L. A., Netea, M. G., & Van Crevel, R. (2011). Innate immune recognition of Mycobacterium tuberculosis. *Clinical & Developmental Immunology, 2011*, 405310.

Korbel, D. S., Schneider, B. E., & Schaible, U. E. (2008). Innate immunity in tuberculosis: Myths and truth. *Microbes and Infection, 10*, 995–1004.

Kulchavenya, E. (2014). Extrapulmonary tuberculosis: Are statistical reports accurate? *Therapeutic Advances in Infectious Disease, 2*, 61–70.

Kumar, P., Pandya, D., Singh, N., Behera, D., Aggarwal, P., & Singh, S. (2014). Loop-mediated isothermal amplification assay for rapid and sensitive diagnosis of tuberculosis. *The Journal of Infection, 69*, 607–615.

Kunnath-Velayudhan, S., & Gennaro, M. L. (2011). Immunodiagnosis of tuberculosis: A dynamic view of biomarker discovery. *Clinical Microbiology Reviews, 24*, 792–805.

Kunnath-Velayudhan, S., Salamon, H., Wang, H. Y., Davidow, A. L., Molina, D. M., Huynh, V. T., Cirillo, D. M., Michel, G., Talbot, E. A., Perkins, M. D., Felgner, P. L., Liang, X., & Gennaro, M. L. (2010). Dynamic antibody responses to the Mycobacterium tuberculosis proteome. *Proceedings of the National Academy of Sciences of the United States of America, 107*, 14703–14708.

Lu, L. L., Chung, A. W., Rosebrock, T. R., Ghebremichael, M., Yu, W. H., Grace, P. S., Schoen, M. K., Tafesse, F., Martin, C., Leung, V., Mahan, A. E., Sips, M., Kumar, M. P., Tedesco, J., Robinson, H., Tkachenko, E., Draghi, M., Freedberg, K. J., Streeck, H., Suscovich, T. J., Lauffenburger, D. A., Restrepo, B. I., Day, C., Fortune, S. M., & Alter, G. (2016). A functional role for antibodies in tuberculosis. *Cell, 167*, 433–443.e14.

Lyashchenko, K. P., Greenwald, R., Esfandiari, J., Greenwald, D., Nacy, C. A., Gibson, S., Didier, P. J., Washington, M., Szczerba, P., Motzel, S., Handt, L., Pollock, J. M., McNair, J., Andersen, P., Langermans, J. A., Verreck, F., Ervin, S., Ervin, F., & McCombs, C. (2007). PrimaTB STAT-PAK assay, a novel, rapid lateral- flow test for tuberculosis in nonhuman primates. *Clinical and Vaccine Immunology, 14*, 1158–1164.

Lyashchenko, K. P., Grandison, A., Keskinen, K., Sikar-Gang, A., Lambotte, P., Esfandiari, J., Ireton, G. C., Vallur, A., Reed, S. G., Jones, G., Vordermeier, H. M., Stabel, J. R., Thacker, T. C., Palmer, M. V., & Waters, W. R. (2017). Identification of novel antigens recognized by serum antibodies in bovine tuberculosis. *Clinical and Vaccine Immunology, 24*, e00259.

Lyashchenko, K. P., Gortazar, C., Miller, M. A., & Waters, W. R. (2018). Spectrum of antibody profiles in tuberculous elephants, cervids, and cattle. *Veterinary Microbiology, 214*, 89–92.

Marriott, I., & Huet-Hudson, Y. M. (2006). Sexual dimorphism in innate immune responses to infectious organisms. *Immunologic Research, 34*, 177–192.

Mihret, A., Bekele, Y., Bobosha, K., Kidd, M., Aseffa, A., Howe, R., & Walzl, G. (2013). Plasma cytokines and chemokines differentiate between active disease and non-active tuberculosis infection. *The Journal of Infection, 66*, 357–365.

Modlin, R. L., & Bloom, B. R. (2013). TB or not TB: That is no longer the question. *Science Translational Medicine, 5*, 213sr216.

Munro, S. A., Lewin, S. A., Smith, H. J., Engel, M. E., Fretheim, A., & Volmink, J. (2007). Patient adherence to tuberculosis treatment: A systematic review of qualitative research. *PLoS Medicine, 4*, e238.

Nhamoyebonde, S., & Leslie, A. (2014). Biological differences between the sexes and susceptibility to tuberculosis. *The Journal of Infectious Diseases, 209*(Suppl 3), S100–S106.

O'Garra, A., Redford, P. S., McNab, F. W., Bloom, C. I., Wilkinson, R. J., & Berry, M. P. (2013). The immune response in tuberculosis. *Annual Review of Immunology, 31*, 475–527.

Pieters, J. (2008). Mycobacterium tuberculosis and the macrophage: Maintaining a balance. *Cell Host & Microbe, 3*, 399–407.

Pollett, S., Banner, P., O'Sullivan, M. V., & Ralph, A. P. (2016). Epidemiology, diagnosis and management of extra-pulmonary tuberculosis in a low-prevalence country: A four year retrospective study in an Australian Tertiary Infectious Diseases Unit. *PLoS One, 11*, e0149372.

Puri, L., Oghor, C., Denkinger, C. M., & Pai, M. (2016). Xpert MTB/RIF for tuberculosis testing: Access and price in highly privatised health markets. *The Lancet Global Health, 4*, e94–e95.

Ravindran, R., Krishnan, V. V., Khanum, A., Luciw, P. A., & Khan, I. H. (2013). Exploratory study on plasma immunomodulator and antibody profiles in tuberculosis patients. *Clinical and Vaccine Immunology, 20*, 1283–1290.

Ravindran, R., Krishnan, V. V., Dhawan, R., Wunderlich, M. L., Lerche, N. W., Flynn, J. L., Luciw, P. A., & Khan, I. H. (2014). Plasma antibody profiles in non-human primate tuberculosis. *Journal of Medical Primatology, 43*, 59–71.

Rhines, A. S. (2013). The role of sex differences in the prevalence and transmission of tuberculosis. *Tuberculosis (Edinburgh, Scotland), 93*, 104–107.

Riou, C., Perez Peixoto, B., Roberts, L., Ronacher, K., Walzl, G., Manca, C., Rustomjee, R., Mthiyane, T., Fallows, D., Gray, C. M., & Kaplan, G. (2012). Effect of standard tuberculosis treatment on plasma cytokine levels in patients with active pulmonary tuberculosis. *PLoS One, 7*, e36886.

Safianowska, A., Walkiewicz, R., Nejman-Gryz, P., & Grubek-Jaworska, H. (2012). [Two selected commercially based nucleic acid amplification tests for the diagnosis of tuberculosis]. *Pneumonologia i Alergologia Polska, 80*, 6–12.

Sasindran, S. J., & Torrelles, J. B. (2011). Mycobacterium tuberculosis infection and inflammation: What is beneficial for the host and for the bacterium? *Frontiers in Microbiology, 2*, 2.

Sharma, S., & Bose, M. (2001). Role of cytokines in immune response to pulmonary tuberculosis. *Asian Pacific Journal of Allergy and Immunology, 19*, 213–219.

Shete, P. B., Ravindran, R., Chang, E., Worodria, W., Chaisson, L. H., Andama, A., Davis, J. L., Luciw, P. A., Huang, L., Khan, I. H., & Cattamanchi, A. (2017). Evaluation of antibody responses to panels of M. tuberculosis antigens as a screening tool for active tuberculosis in Uganda. *PLoS One, 12*, e0180122.

Singh, S., & Katoch, V. M. (2011). Commercial serological tests for the diagnosis of active tuberculosis in India: Time for introspection. *The Indian Journal of Medical Research, 134*, 583–587.

Steingart, K. R., Henry, M., Laal, S., Hopewell, P. C., Ramsay, A., Menzies, D., Cunningham, J., Weldingh, K., & Pai, M. (2007a). Commercial serological antibody detection tests for the diagnosis of pulmonary tuberculosis: A systematic review. *PLoS Medicine, 4*, e202.

Steingart, K. R., Henry, M., Laal, S., Hopewell, P. C., Ramsay, A., Menzies, D., Cunningham, J., Weldingh, K., & Pai, M. (2007b). A systematic review of commercial serological antibody detection tests for the diagnosis of extrapulmonary tuberculosis. *Thorax, 62*, 911–918.

Steingart, K. R., Dendukuri, N., Henry, M., Schiller, I., Nahid, P., Hopewell, P. C., Ramsay, A., Pai, M., & Laal, S. (2009). Performance of purified antigens for serodiagnosis of pulmonary tuberculosis: A meta-analysis. *Clinical and Vaccine Immunology, 16*, 260–276.

Steingart, K. R., Flores, L. L., Dendukuri, N., Schiller, I., Laal, S., Ramsay, A., Hopewell, P. C., & Pai, M. (2011). Commercial serological tests for the diagnosis of active pulmonary and extrapulmonary tuberculosis: An updated systematic review and meta-analysis. *PLoS Medicine, 8*, e1001062.

Subbian, S. (2015). *Rabbit model of mycobacterial diseases*. Oxfordshire, UK: CAB International.

Walzl, G., Ronacher, K., Hanekom, W., Scriba, T. J., & Zumla, A. (2011). Immunological biomarkers of tuberculosis. *Nature Reviews. Immunology, 11*, 343–354.

Waters, W. R., Vordermeier, H. M., Rhodes, B., Khatri, B., Palmer, M. V., Maggioli, M. F., Thacker, T. C., Nelson, J. T., Thomsen, B. V., Robbe-Austerman, S., Bravo Garcia, D. M., Schoenbaum, M. A., Camacho, M. S., Ray, J. S., Esfandiari, J., Lambotte, P., Greenwald, R., Grandison, A., Sikar-Gang, A., & Lyashchenko, K. P. (2017). Potential for rapid antibody detection to identify tuberculous cattle with non-reactive tuberculin skin test results. *BMC Veterinary Research, 13*, 164.

World Health Organization. (2007). *Use of liquid culture and drug susceptibility testing (DST) in low- and middle-income settings. Expert Group Meeting on the issue of liquid culture*. Geneva: World Health Organization.

World Health Organization. (2010). *WHO endorses new rapid tuberculosis test*. www.who.int/mediacenter/news/releases/2010/tb_test_20101208/en/index.html

World Health Organization. (2013). *Roadmap for childhood tuberculosis*. Geneva: World Health Organization.

World Health Organization. (2015). *Global tuberculosis report*. Geneva: World Health Organization.

World Health Organization. (2016). *Fact sheet: World malaria report 2016*. Geneva: World Health Organization.

World Health Organization. (2017). *Global tuberculosis report*. Geneva: World Health Organization.

Yu, Y., Zhang, Y., Hu, S., Jin, D., Chen, X., Jin, Q., & Liu, H. (2012). Different patterns of cytokines and chemokines combined with IFN-gamma production reflect Mycobacterium tuberculosis infection and disease. *PLoS One, 7*, e44944.

Granulomatous Response to *Mycobacterium tuberculosis* Infection

Afsal Kolloli, Pooja Singh, and Selvakumar Subbian

Introduction

Tuberculosis (TB), a deadly infectious disease of humans caused by *Mycobacterium tuberculosis* (Mtb), continues to be a major health threat worldwide. In 2016, there were about 10 million new cases and 1.8 million deaths attributed to TB (WHO Report 2017). The World Health Organization has estimated that about a third of the world population has asymptomatic latent Mtb infection (LTBI) and about 5–10% of individuals develop symptomatic, active primary TB following initial Mtb-infection. However, in a population, Mtb infection results in a heterogeneous outcome, ranging from complete bacterial clearance to the establishment of LTBI or development of a full-blown disease. Although individuals with LTBI are considered to be asymptomatic and noncontagious, about 10% of these individuals can reactivate to symptomatic active TB in their lifetime dependent upon their immune status. The outcome of Mtb infection in humans is dependent on both the host and pathogen-derived factors, including the infectious dose inhaled, the nature of Mtb, and the status of host immunity at the time of infection (Alcais et al. 2005; Zumla et al. 2013). However, a population that remains asymptomatic or do not display disease-like conditions after exposure to Mtb have a chance of 2–23% to remain uninfected for their lifetime. Thus, an individual exposed to Mtb may prevent the establishment of infection. This supports the notion that host immunity is capable of restricting the onset of infection and/or establishing a strong protective response very early after exposure to Mtb. In most of the individuals with LTBI, the bacteria are thought to be maintained inside the granuloma in a dormant form for many years (Lin and Flynn 2010). Active TB can develop either following initial Mtb infection

A. Kolloli · P. Singh · S. Subbian (✉)
Public Health Research Institute, New Jersey Medical School at Rutgers Biomedical and
Health Sciences, Rutgers University, Newark, NJ, USA
e-mail: subbiase@njms.rutgers.edu

© Springer Nature Switzerland AG 2018

41

V. Venketaraman (ed.), *Understanding the Host Immune Response Against*
Mycobacterium tuberculosis Infection, https://doi.org/10.1007/978-3-319-97367-8_3

(primary-progressive TB) or by reactivation of LTBI (post-primary TB); 30–50% of active TB patients develop cavities in their lungs (Benator et al. 2002). Lung cavity is an immunologically weak host environment and is permissive for profound bacterial replication. Cavity formation is considered as one of the detrimental host processes and is indicative of final stages of TB. Patients with pulmonary cavitary TB are highly contagious and are the major source of disease transmission in the community (Rodrigo et al. 1997).

TB is an ancient disease of humans and over the years, Mtb has evolved with its host; bacterial persistence that contributes to reactivation and reinfection are two major difficulties associated with eradication of this deadly disease, as they ultimately provide space for drug tolerance/resistance and emergence of new drug-resistant strains of Mtb. A key feature of TB pathogenesis is granuloma formation, which has been a subject of intense research for several decades. Although granulomas are thought to protect the host by containing Mtb in a confined area and preventing bacterial dissemination to other parts of the body, it is also likely to act as a safe-harbor for the infecting bacteria to thrive and persist in a niche with a compromised immunity.

This chapter summarizes various cellular events underlying TB pathogenesis and the role of different types of immune cells involved in granuloma formation.

Tuberculosis Pathogenesis and Granuloma Formation

Through sneezing, coughing, talking, singing, and related activities, individuals with active pulmonary TB generate and spread aerosol droplets containing pathogenic Mtb that is capable of infecting new hosts. The inhaled bacilli are primarily engulfed by innate phagocytic cells such as alveolar macrophages, neutrophils, and dendritic cells (DCs) in the lung, where the primary inflammatory response is generated with the release of cytokines and chemokines by the infected phagocytes (Huynh et al. 2011) (Fig. 1). At this level, macrophages engulfing Mtb may be classified into two groups, one which is well-activated and capable of killing the bacteria and the other that is suboptimally or poorly activated and providing a growth niche to this intracellular pathogen.

The pathogen recognition receptors (PRRs) present on innate immune cells, such as macrophages, recognize the pathogen-associated molecular patterns (PAMP) present in Mtb, and play a central role in the initiation of host innate immune response (Akira et al. 2006; Pahari et al. 2017). PRRs are either membrane-bound, such as toll-like receptors (TLRs) and C-type lectins, or cytoplasmic, such as NOD-like receptors (NLRs) and RNA helicase retinoic acid-inducible gene I (RIG-I) receptors (Hossain and Norazmi 2013). Among the various TLRs identified, TLR2, TLR4, and TLR9 have key roles in sensing different mycobacterial antigens. The TLR2 interacts with mycobacterial lipoproteins such as 19-kDa secreted lipoprotein (LpqH), LprA and LprG and phosphatidyl-myo-inositol mannoside and induces a strong pro-inflammatory response by activating myeloid differentiation factor 88

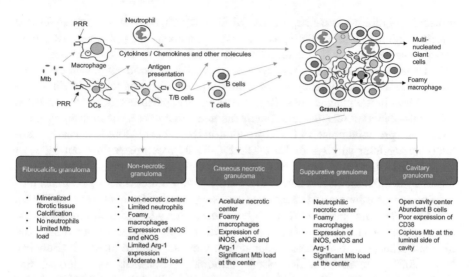

Fig. 1 Architecture and function of granuloma. Following Mtb infection, phagocytes (e.g., macrophage and dendritic cell/DC) uptake the bacteria. The pattern recognition receptors (PRR) present in these antigen presenting cells recognize Mtb antigen that leads to the production of various cytokines and chemokines, which recruit different types of immune cells (neutrophils, T and B cells) to the site of infection to form granuloma. A granuloma is a well-organized cellular structure characterized by the presence of infected macrophages (alveolar, interstitial, foamy, and epithelioid) and DCs that are surrounded by multinucleated giant cells and cuffs of lymphocytes (B and T cells). During disease progression, the granulomas undergo several changes in their structure, immune cell composition and function. Thus, granulomas can be broadly stratified into: (a) fibrocalcific granulomatous nodules, (b) non-necrotic granulomas, (c) caseous necrotic granulomas, and (d) suppurative and cavitary granulomas

(MyD88) and TIR domain-containing adaptor protein (TIRAP) signaling pathways (Quesniaux et al. 2004). Similarly, TLR4 interacts with lipopolysaccharide (LPS) of bacteria and activates MyD88-mediated nuclear factor-κB (NF-κB) signaling pathways, thus inducing the expression of pro-inflammatory cytokines and chemokines (Reiling et al. 2002; Bulut et al. 2005). While TLR9 recognizes CpG DNA of bacteria and promotes pro-inflammatory cytokines production (Hemmi et al. 2000), this receptor can also function cooperatively with TLR2 to induce interferon-gamma (IFN-γ) and IL12p40 production, thus playing a critical role in the development of host-protective immunity to infection (Bafica et al. 2005). Recognition of Mtb antigens by various TLRs also induces maturation of DCs, which migrate from the site of infection to draining lymph nodes and present the antigen to naïve T-cells, thus initiating the adaptive immune response to Mtb infection (Bhatt and Salgame 2007). Moreover, some strains of Mtb activate TLR2, while few others interact with TLR4; this differential stimulation of TLR also leads to differential regulation and/or expression pattern of cytokines and chemokines by the phagocytes and subsequent cellular immune response to the pathogen (Carmona et al. 2013).

There are several types of C-type lectin receptors, such as mannose receptors (MR or CD206) and dendritic cell-specific intercellular adhesion molecule-3-grabbing non-integrin (DC-SIGN/CD209), present on phagocytes that interact with Mtb and mediate phagocytosis. In human macrophages, MR recognizes mannose-capped lipoarabinomannan (ManLAM) of Mtb. It has been proposed that MR-mediated phagocytosis delays the fusion of Mtb-containing phagosome with lysosome, by suppressing the production of phosphatidylinositol-3-phosphate in the phagosomes (Rajaram et al. 2017). Moreover, in Mtb-infected DCs, MR-mediated phagocytosis augments anti-inflammatory response, by interfering with pro-inflammatory IL-12 production (Nigou et al. 2001). This also facilitates intracellular survival of Mtb. The DC-SIGN recognizes different types of PAMPs including LAM, ManLAM, and phosphatidylinositol mannosides (PIMs). Similarly to MR, the interaction of DC-SIGN with ManLAM also modulates pro-inflammatory responses and causes immune suppression (Geijtenbeek et al. 2003). The CD14 receptor plays a crucial role in the monocytic cell differentiation and phagocytosis of Mtb (Lingnau et al. 2007). This receptor recognizes mycobacterial LPS and induces a host-protective innate immune response to infection (Bowdish et al. 2009). Moreover, a decreased pulmonary inflammat ory response was observed in Mtb-infected CD14 knockout mice, which suggests that CD14 has a role in regulating inflammation during chronic pulmonary infection (Wieland et al. 2008). In addition to these cell surface receptors, cytoplasmic receptors can also sense mycobacterial antigens. The NLRs, such as NOD2, can interact with mycobacterial muramyl dipeptide (MDP) and induce pro-inflammatory cytokine production (Divangahi et al. 2008). The NOD2 receptor plays a protective role by sensing the pathogenic Mtb that enters the host cell cytoplasm after rupturing phagosome membrane (Pandey et al. 2009). Thus, the interaction of mycobacterial antigens with specific receptor can activate unique downstream signaling pathway, and their cumulative effect on immune cell activation determines the fate of intracellular Mtb as well as the course of infection towards progressive disease or containment and clearance.

Architecture and Function of Granuloma

Granuloma is a well-organized cellular structure, comprised of infected macrophages (alveolar, interstitial, foamy, and epithelioid), dendritic cells, and neutrophils that are surrounded by multinucleated giant cells, blood-derived macrophages, and cuffs of lymphocytes (T and B cells) (Fig. 1 and Table 1). In a well-organized granuloma, freshly recruited phagocytes and lymphocytes surround the Mtb-infected macrophages. At this stage, the granuloma can act as a physiological barrier and prevent the initial dissemination of infection within and between hosts (Flynn et al. 2011). When a granuloma loses its integrity during early stages and becomes permissive for bacterial growth, then the initial infection progresses into primary active TB. During early stages of infection, an elevated level of pro-inflammatory cytokines, such as TNF-α and IFN-γ produced by immune cells, polarizes the macrophages to a predominantly M1 phenotype that is capable of

Table 1 Immune cells involved in granuloma formation during tuberculosis

No.	Cells	Appearance	Triggered by	Function	References
1.	Epithelial cells and alveolar macrophages	Early stages of infection in the lung parenchyma	Mtb and its components	Recognition and phagocytosis of Mtb	Philips and Ernst (2012)
				Release of cytokines, chemokines and effector molecules	
				Receptors: complement receptor, scavenger receptors, mannose receptor, Dectin-1 and 2, DC-sign, other innate immune sensors	
2.	Multinucleated/Langerhans/giant cells	Mostly at the periphery of granulomatous lesions	TLR-2 dependent activation by mycobacterial lipomannan	Prominent feature of TB granulomas	Sakai et al. (2010)
				Antigen presentation capability	
				Poor phagocytic capacity	
3.	Monocyte derived macrophages and dendritic cells	Early stages of infection and transition of infection to active disease or containment	Mtb and its components	Phagocytosis and antimicrobial response	Uehira et al. (2002); Bodnar et al. (2001)
				Antigen presentation property	
				Migrate to lymph nodes and prime T cell response	
4.	Foamy macrophages	Active disease with necrotic and cavitary granulomas	Mtb and its components, mainly lipids	Accumulation of lipid droplets/bodies	Russell et al. (2009a, b); Welsh et al. (2011)
				Poor phagocytic/anti-microbial/antigen presenting capacity	
5.	Neutrophils	Early stages of infection	Mtb and its components, mainly lipomannan	Phagocytosis and antibacterial response	Zhang et al. (1991); Seiler et al. (2003)
				Initiates inflammatory response	
				Produce MCP1, IL-8 and eicosanoid derivatives	

(continued)

Table 1 (continued)

No.	Cells	Appearance	Triggered by	Function	References
6.	CD4+ T cells	Transition of infection to active disease or containment	Antigen presenting cells stimulated by Mtb antigens	IFNγ production	Ladel et al. (1995); Boselli et al. (2007); Lockhart et al. (2006)
				MHC-II presentation	
				Activation of macrophages	
				Organize/maintain granulomas	
	CD8+ T cells	Chronic infection/disease	Antigen presenting cells stimulated by Mtb antigens	XCL-1 production	
				Negatively regulates IFNγ production	
				Cytotoxic effects on infected cells	
7.	B cells	Transition of infection to active disease or containment Chronic disease	Mycobacterial antigens	Differentiate into plasma cells	Maglione et al. (2007)
				Generate Mtb antigen specific antibodies	
				Enhance CD4+ T cell response	

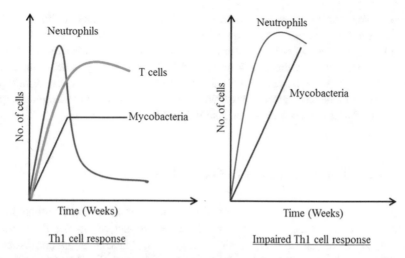

Fig. 2 Host immune response during Mtb infection. Th1 immune response plays a critical role during granuloma formation and restricts bacterial growth. Optimal onset of Th1 response along with protracted neutrophil infiltration enables containment of bacteria in the granulomas (left panel), while increased infiltration of neutrophils to the site of infection and impaired Th1 response increase inflammation and tissue destruction that contribute to elevated bacterial load (right panel)

controlling Mtb growth and replication, through their antimicrobial effector functions. In addition, M1 macrophages can efficiently present Mtb antigens to T cells, which mount a host-protective Th1 type immunity by recruiting and activating more innate and adaptive immune cells with a pro-inflammatory phenotype. These cells surround the infected macrophages at the center of granuloma and limit the spread of Mtb (Chakravarty et al. 2008). Thus, the quality and quantity of immune response elicited by M1 macrophages, followed by immune cell recruitment and actvation of CD4⁺ and CD8⁺ T cells, mark the type of immune response generated in a granuloma (Fig. 2). However, as the disease progresses, the immune environment changes and the macrophages are more permissive to Mtb growth and polarized toward an anti-inflammatory M2 phenotype, marked with elevated IL-4 and IL-10 production. This facilitates establishment of a Th2 type immune environment with increased IL-2, IL-4, and I-10 production by immune cells; all these events are also associated with elevated lipid metabolism that contributes to formation of foamy macrophages (Kim et al. 2010).

During active disease, the Mtb-infected macrophages at the center of granulomas undergo necrosis that results in the accumulation of caseum, a creamy and acellular region, in which Mtb can survive extracellularly. Uncontrolled necrosis of infected host cells contributes to granuloma rupture and dissemination of pathogen to neighboring tissues facilitating secondary granuloma formation; these are seen in the lungs of about 20% of active TB cases, while reactivation of Mtb from quiescent granulomas contributes to active lung disease in about 80% of cases (Frieden et al. 2003). Even though granulomas are thought to restrict Mtb growth and dissemination, it is also suggested to promote bacterial persistence, which is a potential reservoir for future disease reactivation (Davis and Ramakrishnan 2009). Mycobacterial components are known to stimulate IL-10 secretion thereby suppressing Th1 response (Davis and Ramakrishnan 2009) and promoting M2 macrophage polarization with the development of lipid-rich, foamy macrophages and giant cells (Lugo-Villarino et al. 2012). This phenomenon suggests that granulomas can serve as a niche to support Mtb growth and/or survival by providing host lipids as a carbon source (Davis and Ramakrishnan 2009).

Structural Transformation of Granuloma

The granuloma physically maintains the bulk of Mtb in the organs of infected individuals. However, during progression of infection into active disease, the granulomas undergo several changes, mediated through the immune cells that constitute the granulomas, including structural transformation and metabolic shift (Russell et al. 2009a, b; Cadena et al. 2017). There is a strong positive correlation between the structural organization of granuloma and the extent of disease progression (Marino et al. 2011). While solid granulomas, marked with well-activated immune cells and no necrosis can effectively control Mtb growth and infection, cavitary granulomas with necrotic center are permissive for bacterial growth and disease progression. This suggests that any host debilitating conditions, such as immune deficiency (e.g., HIV infection, immune suppressive treatment) or metabolic disorder (e.g., diabetics) can alter the granuloma's integrity and significantly affect the disease status. According to their structural organization, granulomas can be broadly stratified into: (a) fibro-calcific nodules, (b) non-necrotic, (c) caseous necrotic, (d) suppurative, and (e) cavitary granulomas (Mattila et al. 2013; Cadena et al. 2017). The fibro-calcific nodules are usually found in individuals with LTBI and believed to have a host protective role in controlling Mtb infection from transmission. These are usually smaller, healing-type granulomas (a.k.a. Ghon's focus), characterized by mineralized fibrotic tissue and calcification at the center; both these processes can reduce bacterial survival and the probability of disease reactivation (Lin et al. 2009). In these granulomas, the fibrotic center is surrounded by large numbers of lymphocytes, macrophages (predominantly CD163+), and a restricted number of neutrophils (Lin et al. 2012).

The non-necrotic granulomas are highly cellular and characterized by the absence of cellular necrosis at the center, which is surrounded by both CD68+ and CD163+ macrophages. Limited number of neutrophils, abundant HAM56+ foamy macrophages, elevated proportion of epithelioid macrophages that strongly express iNOS and eNOS, and a relatively low frequency of Arg-1 expressing monocytes/macrophages are also observed in these granulomas. The caseous necrotic and suppurative granulomas have almost related features with a necrotic center. In caseous necrotic granuloma, the necrotic region is acellular with moderate number of neutrophils, whereas large number of neutrophils are present in the vicinity of necrotic center in suppurative granulomas (Mattila et al. 2013). In these granulomas, both CD68+ and

CD163+ macrophages are distributed in and around the lymphocyte cuff. While the CD163+ macrophages are predominantly present in the peripheral region, HAM56+ foamy macrophages are abundant mainly at the rim of necrotic center. Both iNOS and Arg-1 are expressed abundantly throughout the necrotic granuloma, including lymphocytic cuff and the periphery of necrotic region. It is suggested that the ratio between iNOS and Arg-1 expression levels might play an important role in the structural transformation of granuloma and subsequent disease progression (Mattila et al. 2013; Kramnik and Beamer 2016).

Cavitation of granulomas in the lungs is a prelude to transmission of infection/ Mtb within and between host(s). The luminal wall of cavitary lesions have copious number of Mtb actively proliferating extracellularly; since cavitary lesions in pulmonary tuberculosis open into airways and enable aerosol generation, they facilitate disease transmission (Kaplan et al. 2003). These lesions are thought to be manifestations of secondary (post-primary) tuberculosis, marked by elevated levels of regulatory T cells (Tregs) and DEC-205+ DCs (Welsh et al. 2011). Histologically, cavitary granulomas are characterized by severe tissue inflammation, suboptimal activation of innate and adaptive immune cells, and accumulation of B cells in the granuloma (Subbian et al. 2011). The cellular and immunological responses in cavitary lesions are also significantly different from non-necrotic and fibro-capsular lung lesions (Ulrichs et al. 2005). It has been suggested that differential regulation of local immune response at the site of infection determines the evolution of granulomas. Therefore, in patients with active pulmonary TB and in nonhuman primates and rabbit models of TB, remarkable heterogeneity in granulomas can be seen within the same lung that correlates with diseas progression or control of infection (Subbian et al. 2011; Ulrichs et al. 2005; Cadena et al. 2017).

Role of Cytokines in Granuloma Formation

The interaction of Mtb with PRRs of innate immune cells induces production of both pro- and anti-inflammatory cytokines and chemokines. While a pro-inflammatory response further activates the innate and adaptive immune cells and mediates granuloma formation, an anti-inflammatory response dampens inflammation and counteracts the effects of pro-inflammatory responses to avoid tissue damage. Although the former response is thought to be protective against Mtb infection, a delicate balance between pro- and anti-inflammatory responses is crucial for effective control of Mtb infection and tissue destruction (Domingo-Gonzalez et al. 2016). TNF-α is a key pro-inflammatory cytokine, produced by the cells of innate and adaptive immunity following Mtb infection, and plays key roles during granuloma formation and maintenance. It induces the production of chemokines such as CCL5 (RANTES), CXCL9 (MIG), and CXCL10 (IP-10) from various types of immune cells (Akira et al. 2006). These chemokines bind to respective receptors expressed on the surface of activated T cells, B cells, macrophages, and neutrophils and mediate extravasation of leukocytes to the primary site of infection to form the granuloma. TNF-α also maintains granuloma integrity that prevents reactivation and dissemination of Mtb (Chakravarty et al. 2008). In LTBI individuals, neutralization of TNF-α resulted in reactivation of symptomatic, active TB (Keane et al. 2001). This observation has also been confirmed in mouse and rabbit models of Mtb infection, in which treatment with anti-TNF-α antibodies suppressed host immunity, exacerbated disease severity, and bacillary load (Koo et al. 2011; Tsenova et al. 2014). These studies underline the protective role of TNF-α and the importance of granuloma integrity in TB.

Mycobacterial components are presented through infected macrophages and DC to the cells of the adaptive immunity, such as CD4+ and CD8+ T cells, Treg, and natural killer (NK) cells. DCs with engulfed Mtb can migrate from the lungs to regional lymph nodes to prime naive CD4+ and CD8+ T cells that ultimately become effector and memory subsets and play distinct roles in TB pathogenesis (O'Garra et al. 2013). In the granuloma, CD4+ T cells at the periphery of infected macrophages predominantly secrete interferon-γ (IFN-γ), a key pro-inflammatory cytokine, which activates the antimicrobial activities of phagocytes and facilitates antigen-specific T cell response (Cooper 2009). In addition, IFN-γ regulates systemic and local (lung) inflammation by inhibiting IL-17 production and neutrophil infiltration at the site of infection (Nandi and Behar 2011). In contrast, type I IFNs, such as IFN-α and IFN-β, are thought to inhibit the IFN-γ-mediated antimicrobial processes as well as the recruitment of CD4+ and CD8+ cells to the granuloma while promoting neutrophils infiltration to the site of infection (Ordway et al. 2007; Berry et al. 2010).

Cytokines that belong to the IL-1 family, such as IL-1α, IL-1β, and IL-18, can also initiate a pro-inflammatory response during Mtb infection. IL-1α has been shown to induce the production of IL-6 in human lung fibroblast, which activates host-protective effects on Mtb-infected macrophages; whereas IL-1β restricts intracellular Mtb growth in macrophages by enhancing phagosome maturation, autophagy, and production of antimicrobial peptides such as β-defensin 4 (Suwara et al. 2014; Master et al. 2008; Liu et al. 2009; Verway et al. 2013). IL-18 is known to induce pro-inflammatory IFN-γ production from T cells and thus plays a protective role against Mtb infection (Kinjo et al. 2002). Similarly, IL-6 produced by phagocytes upon Mtb infection plays a critical role in the onset of early inflammatory response (Law et al. 1996; Hoheisel et al. 1998). This cytokine regulates neutrophil infiltration (Fielding et al. 2008) and mediates differentiation and maintenance of Th17 cells, which contribute to establishment of an acute inflammatory response during Mtb infection (Jones and Vignali 2011). IL-12 is an important host-protective cytokine against Mtb infection and has vital roles in both innate and adaptive immune responses. IL-12 (IL-12p70) is composed of two subunits, IL-12p35 and IL-12/23p40, and is mainly secreted by Mtb-activated DCs. This cytokine is also a potent inducer of IFN-γ producing T cells, which are important to control Mtb infection (Cooper et al. 2011). It has been shown that infection of DCs by Mtb can trigger IL-12p40 secretion through TLR2 or TLR9 signaling pathways (Bafica et al. 2005). In addition, IL-12p40 regulates adaptive immune response and is required for DC migration and T cell priming in the lymph nodes during Mtb infection

(Khader et al. 2006). The importance of IL-12 receptors is highlighted in recent studies, which show that mutations in the IL-12 receptor β1 (IL-12Rβ1) abrogate cellular immune response to IL-12 and compromise protective immunity to Mtb infection. Similarly, autosomal recessive IL-12Rβ1 deficiency in adults and children has been shown to result in severe disseminated forms of TB (Boisson-Dupuis et al. 2011; Tabarsi et al. 2011).

During Mtb infection, a subset of T cells, namely the Th17 cells, mainly produces pro-inflammatory cytokine IL-17, which promotes granuloma formation and plays a significant role in restricting Mtb growth (Okamoto Yoshida et al. 2010). IL-17 has been shown to induce IFN-γ and IL-12 secretion by macrophages and DCs that enhance host-protective Th1 immune responses (Lin et al. 2009). In addition, IL-17 induces the expression of chemokine CXCL13 and promotes the accumulation of CXCR5+ T cells at the site of infection (Gopal et al. 2013). These T cells are long-living and contribute to improved protection offered by BCG vaccination against Mtb infection (Desel et al. 2011; Lindenstrom et al. 2012). However, studies have also shown that IL-17 mediates excessive neutrophil recruitment, which contributes to elevated tissue inflammation and disease pathology during Mtb infection (Cruz et al. 2010). Therefore, it appears that fine-tuning of Th17 cell activation and IL-17 production is important for optimal host protection to Mtb infection. Another cytokine that plays key roles in the differentiation and maintenance of Th17 cells and development of B cell follicles during Mtb infection is IL-23 (Khader et al. 2011). This cytokine also induces the development of IFN-γ producing Th1 cells and proliferation of memory T cells in response to Mtb infection (Wozniak et al. 2006). Following Mtb infection, CD4+ cells, NK cells, and other lymphoid cells also express IL-22, a cytokine that stimulates production of antimicrobial peptides, such as β-defensin and lipocalin (McAleer and Kolls 2014). A higher level of IL-22 is reported in pulmonary TB granulomas (Matthews et al. 2011), where it activates macrophages and restricts intracellular Mtb growth by promoting phagolysosome fusion (Dhiman et al. 2014). In addition, IL-22 has been shown to mediate antigen-specific T cell responses, while suppressing the expansion of infection-induced Tregs, thus contributing positively to vaccine-mediated protective immunity to TB (Dhiman et al. 2009).

In contrast to the Th1 type cells, the Th2 and Tregs cells express key immune-regulatory cytokines, such as IL-4, IL-5, IL-10, IL-13, and TGF-β. These cytokines inhibit Th1 responses and regulate inflammatory response during Mtb infection. IL-4 downregulates the expression of inducible nitric oxide synthase (iNOS) and TLR2, thus contributing to dampening of macrophage activation and disease progression (Gordon 2003; Krutzik et al. 2003). However, increased expression of IL-4 also promotes necrosis of immune cells in the granuloma that facilitate extracellular bacterial replication, disease progression, and lung cavitation (Mazzarella et al. 2003; Bezuidenhout et al. 2009). IL-10 is another important immune-regulatory cytokine induced during Mtb infection. This cytokine exerts anti-inflammatory effect via STAT3-dependent pathway that inhibits macrophage activation (Cassatella et al. 1999; Moore et al. 2001; O'Leary et al. 2011). IL-10 also suppresses T cell proliferation and inhibits pro-inflammatory Th1 and Th17 responses during Mtb infection (Kumar et al. 2013). Similarly, IL-13 promotes Mtb survival by downregulating IFN-γ-induced autophagy in infected phagocytes (Harris et al. 2007). Increased expression of IL-13 reduces the frequency of IFN-γ and IL-17-expressing CD4+ T cells and augments necrotic cell death in TB granulomas (Heitmann et al. 2014). Mycobacterial membrane components, such as lipoarabino-mannan (LAM), can induce the production of TGF-β by monocytes and DCs at the sites of infection (Toossi et al. 1995; Condos et al. 1998). This anti-inflammatory cytokine can suppress Th1 immune response by dampening IFN-γ production, antigen presentation, and pro-inflammatory cytokine production in Mtb-infected macrophages (Toossi and Ellner 1998). It has been shown that the combined induction of IL-10, TGF-β, TGF-β receptor 1 (RI) and RII expression can down-modulate the host immune response to Mtb infection and favors subsequent disease progression and bacterial growth (Bonecini-Almeida et al. 2004).

Role of Chemokines in Granuloma Formation

Several chemokines have been reported to mediate the early migration of immune cells to facilitate granuloma formation at the site of Mtb infection (Flynn and Chan 2005). These chemokines are classified as CXC or alpha, CC or beta, C or gamma, and CX3C or delta, based on the location of cysteine residues. Chemokines exert their function through interaction with respective receptors, which are members of the G1 protein coupled receptors (GPCR). The CC-type chemokines, such as monocyte chemoattractant protein-1 (MCP-1/CCL2), macrophage inflammatory protein-1α (MIP-1α/CCL3) and MIP-1β (CCL4) regulated upon activation, normal T cell expressed and secreted (RANTES/CCL5), as well as CXC-type chemokines, such as IL-8, monokine induced by gamma interferon (MIG/CXCL9), interferon gamma inducible protein-10 (IP-10/CXCL10), and stromal cell derived factor-1 (SDF-1/CXCL12), have been demonstrated to play key roles during Mtb infection and granuloma formation (Domingo-Gonzalez et al. 2016).

The CC-chemokine MCP-1 is one of the most potent chemoattractants of immune cells and activator of monocytes and plays an important role in regulating the host-pathogen interactions during Mtb infection. This chemokine is primarily secreted by monocytes, macrophages, and DCs, and it attracts both Th1 and Th2 cells to the site of infection (Siveke and Hamann 1998). However, it has been reported that MCP-1 enhances polarization of naïve T cells to Th2 cells, which can lead to an inefficient control of Mtb infection by the immune cells (Hussain et al. 2011). MIP-1α and MIP-1β are potent chemoattractants/activators of pro-inflammatory cells in the granuloma (Collins and Kaufmann 2001; Algood et al. 2003). These chemokines can also activate granulocytes, such as neutrophils and eosinophils, which lead to acute inflammation (Hsieh et al. 2008). While MIP-1α can induce the production of cytokines such as TNF-α, IL-1β, and IL-6, MIP-1β has been shown to modulate CCL3-induced TNF-α production in macrophages (Fahey et al. 1992). It has been shown that Mtb-infected human alveolar macrophages induce the production of RANTES, which helps to reduce intracellular Mtb growth (Saukkonen et al. 2002). This chemokine can attract immune cells to the site of infection and promote granuloma formation. CCL5 is another host-protective chemokine, which mediates recruitment of IFN-γ-producing, antigen-specific T cells expressing CCR5, a receptor for CCL5. Thus, CCL5 limits the intracellular survival of Mtb and contributes to host protection (Vesosky et al. 2010). In addition, coordinated expression/function of CCL5, perforin, and granulysin in CD8+ T cells facilitates killing of Mtb within infected macrophages (Stegelmann et al. 2005).

The CXC-chemokine, IL-8, is produced by epithelial cells, monocytes, macrophages, and fibroblasts during Mtb infection. This chemokine is an important neutrophil chemoattractant and reported to have a significant role in the inflammatory response and control of Mtb infection (O'Kane et al. 2007). Elevated serum levels of IL-8 were noted in patients with active pulmonary TB, which decreased to basal levels following successful anti-TB chemotherapy treatment (Almeida Cde et al. 2009). Thus, IL-8 has been suggested as a potent biomarker of TB to measure disease severity and treatment efficacy. The IFN-γ inducible chemokines, MIG and IP-10 (CXCL10), are chemotactic for NK cells and activated T lymphocytes. It has been shown that the expression of MIG enhances the recruitment of IFN-γ producing CD4+ T cells to the granulomas, which helps to restrict bacterial growth (Khader et al. 2007). During Mtb infection, IP-10 acts as an immune-inflammatory mediator and plays an important role in the granuloma formation by recruiting activated CXCR3+ T cells to the infection site (Agostini et al. 1998; Zhang et al. 2004). In addition, most of the peripheral CXCR3+ T cells express CD45RO (memory T cells), which is implicated in binding of lymphocytes to endothelial cells. Elevated levels of IP-10 has been detected in the plasma/sera of patients with active TB as well as subclinical and LTBI cases; although this chemokine has been suggested as a promising diagnostic marker for active TB (Strzelak et al. 2012). The stromal cell derived factor-1 (SDF-1) is a homeostatic CXC-type chemokine that is involved in myelopoiesis, B-lymphopoiesis, and localization and retention of progenitor cells in bone marrow as well as in organ development (Moser and Loetscher 2001). Increased levels of SDF-1 have been reported in the plasma of patients with active pulmonary TB (Shalekoff and Tiemessen 2003). A recent study has also shown that during Mtb infection, SDF-1 attracts circulating CXCR4+ B cells to the pleural space, thus playing an important role in B cell trafficking to the site of infection (Feng et al. 2011). Moreover, SDF-1 has been suggested as a diagnostic marker for differentiating TB pleurisy from other forms of TB (Kohmo et al. 2012). Thus, chemokine-mediated recruitment of immune cells to the site infection plays central role in the granuloma formation and disease pathogenesis in TB.

B Cell Response in Tuberculosis

Adaptive immune response in TB, elicited by lymphocytes upon Mtb infection of the host, can be broadly divided into T cell-mediated cellular immunity and B cell-mediated humoral immunity. Although T cell-mediated cellular immune response is crucial in controlling Mtb infection and regulating granuloma formation/maturation, several studies have shown that B cells and their antibody-mediated humoral immune response can also impact the host responses against Mtb infection (Jacobs et al. 2016). A recent study reported that B cell responses are dysregulated in patients with active and latent TB, and this impairment was not observed in individuals after anti-TB treatment (Joosten et al. 2016). This study also shows that B cells augment the effector functions of cellular immune response mediated by T cells. The B cells present in TB granulomas mediate several immune processes such as antigen presentation to T cells, Mtb-specific antibody production, and promoting the development of Th1 response by inducing IL-12 and IFN-γ production (Kozakiewicz et al. 2013; Chan et al. 2014; Bao et al. 2014). Antibodies to Mtb, secreted by the B cells, are thought to be involved in the neutralization of toxin, opsonization, and modulation of complement-mediated lysis. Moreover, IgG antibody specific to mycobacterial antigen has been found in the plasma of TB patients (Daniel et al. 1981). The antibody-mediated immune response is more prominent in the granulomas during disease progression, where bacteria replicate extracellularly in the necrotic material. It is proposed that anti-Mtb antibodies can prevent the establishment or dissemination of Mtb infection by hampering the bacterial adhesion to phagocytes (Schlesinger et al. 1994). For example, in macrophages, the FcR-mediated phagocytosis of Mtb was shown to enhance phagolysosomal fusion and myco-peptide presentation to T cells, thus augmenting the Th1 response (Maglione et al. 2008; Guilliams et al. 2014). In addition, the pre-coating of bacilli with anti-LAM antibodies has been shown to enhance phagolysosomal fusion and to increase the abundance of IFN-γ-expressing CD4+ and CD8+ T cells (de Valliere et al. 2005; Kumar et al. 2015). In addition, higher levels of anti-Mtb isotype IgG3 antibodies have been shown to be associated with preventio of LTBI reactivation in high-risk individuals (Encinales et al. 2010). Similarly, passive administration of Mtb-specific monoclonal antibodies as well as human gamma globulin has been shown to provide a protective effect against Mtb infection (Hamasur et al. 2004; Olivares et al. 2009; Balu et al. 2011). Furthermore, B cells can help to regulate inflammation in the infected tissue by secreting anti-inflammatory cytokines, such as TGF-b, IL-4, and IL-33, and by regulating Th1 and Th17 response (Chan et al. 2014). Moreover, B cells regulate neutrophil infiltration at the site of infection by modulating IL-17 response and thus help to prevent exacerbated inflammatory response during Mtb infection (Kozakiewicz et al. 2013).

Metabolic Shift in Granulomas

Infections by pathogens and/or environmental stresses, such as limited nutrient availability, hypoxia, and low pH, are capable of modulating the central metabolism of immune cells that can alter the protective host response and contribute to disease progression. A metabolic shift toward enhanced glycolysis with diminished oxygen consumption is a key feature of immune cells in TB granulomas (Shi et al. 2016). Mtb infection has been shown to modulate the host metabolome by increasing glucose oxidation and lipid peroxidation that ultimately lead to accumulation of several metabolites such as gluconic acid, lactone, glutaric acid, butanal, and ethane. Importantly, presence of these metabolic intermediates has been confirmed in the sputum samples of patients with active pulmonary TB (du Preez and Loots 2013). Upon Mtb infection, the metabolic reprogramming is mainly found in classically activated, pro-inflammatory M1 macrophages, immunogenic DCs, and activated T cells but not in anti-inflammatory M2 macrophages and tolerogenic DCs. The metabolic shift in TB granuloma has similar characteristics of the Warburg effect reported in cancer cells, which contributes to the increased production of nitric oxide and pro-inflammatory cytokines (Shi et al. 2016; Kiran et al. 2016). During Mtb infection, several genes associated with the Warburg effect (e.g., H+-ATPase, glucose transporters, and glycolytic enzymes such as hexokinase, phosphofructokinase, phosphoglycerate kinase, enolase, ADP-dependent glucose kinase, and lactate dehydrogenase) were shown to be upregulated (Shi et al. 2016). In addition, induction of Warburg effect in the host immune cells is also associated with corresponding increase in the expression of hypoxia-inducible factor-1 alpha (HIF-1 α), which plays a key regulatory role during infection and inflammation (Semenza 2010). In addition, HIF-1α regulates the expression of pro-inflammatory cytokines and differentiation of Th17 cells (Dang et al. 2011). In TB granulomas, HIF-1α-induced Warburg effect is associated with activation of pyruvate kinase M2 (PKM2), a key regulator of glycolysis. Translocation of PKM2 to the nucleus and its interaction with HIF-1α activates expression of pro-inflammatory cytokines, such as IL-1β and the glycolytic enzymes (Palsson-McDermott et al. 2015).

In addition to the shift in glucose metabolism, altered lipid metabolism has also been reported in the immune cells of TB granulomas. Mtb upregulates expression of several host genes involved in lipid sequestration and metabolism such as adipophilin (ADFP), acyl Co-A synthase long-chain family member 1 (ACSL1), and prosaposin (PSAP) in caseous granulomas (Kim et al. 2010). Similarly, an increased production of cholesterol (CHO), cholesterol ester (CE), triacylglycerol (TAG), and lactosylceramide (LacCer) has been reported in TB granulomas (Chatterjee et al. 1997; Garner et al. 2002). This Mtb-induced lipid sequestration can lead to the accumulation of lipid droplets in the cytoplasm and other organelles of macrophages and subsequent foamy macrophage formation (Daniel et al. 2011). Mtb can persist and replicate in foamy macrophages and their presence is an indication of degenerative granuloma and caseous necrosis (Tan and Russell 2015). Furthermore, Mtb can utilize host-derived lipid intermediates, such as TAG as its carbon source for growth and replication (Pandey and Sassetti 2008). Thus, altered immune cell metabolism during Mtb infection can augment bacterial outgrowth and necrosis of granuloma and a delicate balance in host immunometabolism is crucial for an effective host-protective response.

Targeting Granulomas as a Therapeutic Approach for TB

Although granuloma plays a significant role in the prevention of initial stage of Mtb infection towards progressive disease, presence of multiple types of granulomas, ranging from cavitary to necrotic and non-necrotic lesions, within the lungs of active TB patients questions its protective role. Moreover, granulomas, by virtue of their tight-knit cellular structure with fibrotic rims, can be refractory to antibiotics penetration into their necrotic center with caseum, where Mtb thrives; this contributes to prolonged duration of anti-TB treatment (at least 6 months for drug-sensitive pulmonary TB). This also suggests that additional host-directed therapeutic strategy that can modulate the structure (e.g., integrity, vascularization) and function (inflammation, metabolism) of granulomas can be used to enhance the efficacy of existing anti-TB drugs (Kolloli and Subbian 2017). Previous findings show promising trend in this approach. For example, TNF-α plays a significant role in the formation of granuloma and maintenance of its integrity; neutralization of TNF-α with antibody (e.g., Enbrel) treatment leads to disruption of granuloma integrity and enhances antibiotic penetration that augments bacterial clearance and reduces lung pathology (Chakravarty et al. 2008; Bourigault et al. 2013). Similarly, blocking of TNF-α using etanercept during initial stages of TB treatment was shown to accelerate sputum culture conversion and elevate the number of CD4+ T cells by 25% in patients with HIV-associated TB (Wallis et al. 2004). These findings suggest that granuloma integrity is a critical factor for bacterial survival and proliferation, and therapeutic agents that can perturb granuloma structure have the potential to be used as adjunct drug with standard antibiotics to promote efficient bacterial clearance, improve treatment efficacy, and shorten the duration of therapy.

Recently, pharmacological agents that either promote or inhibit angiogenesis have been reported to augment TB treatment. In this strategy, the host vascular endothelial growth factor (VEGF) and angiopoietins (Ang) were targeted. These molecules are potent angiogenic factors and are essential for the growth and proliferation of endothelial cells. Moreover, VEGF and Ang are abundantly expressed in pulmonary TB granulomas (Datta et al. 2015) and elevated levels of these molecules have been reported in patients with active pulmonary TB, compared to healthy controls (Kumar et al. 2016). The increased expression of VEGF and Ang also promotes abnormal, leaky, and dysfunctional blood vessel formation around the granulomatous area. This creates a hypoxic microenvironment in the granuloma that impairs normal immune response and favors Mtb persistence (Osherov and Ben-Ami 2016). Recently, the ability of an anti-VEGF antibody (Bevacizumab) or treatment with SU5416 (tyrosine kinase receptor), and pazopanib (VEGFR inhibitor) in normalizing the vascular structure of granulomas was investigated (Oehlers et al. 2015; Datta et al. 2015). Results from these studies show successful neutralization of VEGR function that reduced hypoxia and facilitated anti-TB drug penetration and killing of Mtb in the granuloma (Oehlers et al. 2015; Datta et al. 2015).

In addition to controlling angiogenesis, recent research also focused on an alternative strategy, which promotes normal angiogenesis in the granulomas to augment anti-TB treatment with antibiotics. Since granulomas are limited in their blood supply and circulation, restoring normal angiogenesis might improve the immune response and delivery of anti-TB drugs. The lack of VEGF in the sera of patients with active, cavitary pulmonary TB supports this approach (Abe et al. 2001). Therefore, any therapeutic approach that promotes expression of angiogenic growth factors such as VEGF, epidermal growth factors, transforming growth factor, platelet-derived growth factor, fibroblast growth factor, and hypoxia-inducible factor can be used to improve the clinical outcome of current anti-TB treatment. Since hormones involved in glucose homeostasis promote angiogenesis, targeting these hormones can be another promising approach to improve TB treatment (Cun et al. 2015). For example, exenatide, an agonist of the glucagon-like peptide-1 receptor that enhances angiogenesis in endothelial cells, has been reported to promote angiogenesis in TB granuloma (Aronis et al. 2013). Although clinical intervention to restore and normalize vascular structure might enhance the efficacy of anti-TB chemotherapy, more preclinical studies are required to assess the beneficial role of targeting granuloma integrity and restoring tissue angiogenesis for better delivery of anti-TB drugs.

Summary and Conclusion

To summarize, following successful entry into the lungs, pathogenic Mtb interacts with host cell receptors present on phagocytic cells in the lungs. This leads to engulfment of the pathogen and secretion of several pro-inflammatory molecules, which aid in the extravasation of various immune cells from the circulation to the site of infection and initiate granuloma formation. With time, the granuloma is packed with various leukocytes and confined to a defined area in the lungs. These host cells produce a plethora of cytokines/chemokines that shapes the quality of immune response prevailing in the granuloma. In general, a pro-inflammatory Th1 response is considered as host protective while an anti-inflammatory Th2 response is considered as counter-protective against Mtb infection; although a delicate balance between Th1 and Th2 response is crucial for optimal control of infection. Within the granuloma, the bacteria are either contained or proliferate and disseminate, depending on the nature of the bacteria and the immune environment prevailing in the granuloma. In general, during early stages of infection, granulomas wall off replication/dissemination of bacteria/disease and play a host-protective role. During progression of infection to active disease, the lung granulomas undergo structural changes and deteriorate to develop central caseous necrosis. At this stage, Mtb actively multiplies extracellularly within the granuloma that can undergo structural changes leading to lung cavitation. In addition, immune cells present in the granuloma can adopt a metabolic shift with enhanced glycolysis and altered lipid metabolism. Considering the limitations associated with current antibiotic-based therapy, adjunct host-directed therapeutic modalities, such as those that target granuloma, is a novel and new treatment approach for TB. In this approach, the structure and/or immune cell function of granulomas can be modulated to increase better anti-TB drug delivery and/or accessibility for efficient bacteriall killing and control of infection. This strategy can improve the efficacy of existing anti-TB drugs, help to reduce the duration therapy, and elevate the quality of clinical outcome following treatment of patients with TB.

References

Abe, Y., Nakamura, M., Oshika, Y., Hatanaka, H., Tokunaga, T., Ohkubo, Y., et al. (2001). Serum levels of vascular endothelial growth factor and cavity formation in active pulmonary tuberculosis. *Respiration, 68*(5), 496–500.

Agostini, C., Cassatella, M., Zambello, R., Trentin, L., Gasperini, S., Perin, A., et al. (1998). Involvement of the IP-10 chemokine in sarcoid granulomatous reactions. *Journal of Immunology, 161*(11), 6413–6420.

Akira, S., Uematsu, S., & Takeuchi, O. (2006). Pathogen recognition and innate immunity. *Cell, 124*(4), 783–801.

Alcais, A., Fieschi, C., Abel, L., & Casanova, J. L. (2005). Tuberculosis in children and adults: Two distinct genetic diseases. *The Journal of Experimental Medicine, 202*(12), 1617–1621.

Algood, H. M., Chan, J., & Flynn, J. L. (2003). Chemokines and tuberculosis. *Cytokine & Growth Factor Reviews, 14*(6), 467–477.

Almeida Cde, S., Abramo, C., Alves, C. C., Mazzoccoli, L., Ferreira, A. P., & Teixeira, H. C. (2009). Anti-mycobacterial treatment reduces high plasma levels of CXC-chemokines detected in active tuberculosis by cytometric bead array. *Memórias do Instituto Oswaldo Cruz, 104*(7), 1039–1041.

Aronis, K. N., Chamberland, J. P., & Mantzoros, C. S. (2013). GLP-1 promotes angiogenesis in human endothelial cells in a dose-dependent manner, through the Akt, Src and PKC pathways. *Metabolism, 62*(9), 1279–1286.

Bafica, A., Scanga, C. A., Feng, C. G., Leifer, C., Cheever, A., & Sher, A. (2005). TLR9 regulates Th1 responses and cooperates with TLR2 in mediating optimal resistance to Mycobacterium tuberculosis. *The Journal of Experimental Medicine, 202*(12), 1715–1724.

Balu, S., Reljic, R., Lewis, M. J., Pleass, R. J., McIntosh, R., van Kooten, C., et al. (2011). A novel human IgA monoclonal antibody protects against tuberculosis. *Journal of Immunology, 186*(5), 3113–3119.

Bao, Y., Liu, X., Han, C., Xu, S., Xie, B., Zhang, Q., et al. (2014). Identification of IFN-gamma-producing innate B cells. *Cell Research, 24*(2), 161–176.

Benator, D., Bhattacharya, M., Bozeman, L., Burman, W., Cantazaro, A., Chaisson, R., et al. (2002). Rifapentine and isoniazid once a week versus rifampicin and isoniazid twice a week for treatment of drug-susceptible pulmonary tuberculosis in HIV-negative patients: A randomised clinical trial. *Lancet, 360*(9332), 528–534.

Berry, M. P., Graham, C. M., McNab, F. W., Xu, Z., Bloch, S. A., Oni, T., et al. (2010). An interferon- inducible neutrophil-driven blood transcriptional signature in human tuberculosis. *Nature, 466*(7309), 973–977.

Bezuidenhout, J., Roberts, T., Muller, L., van Helden, P., & Walzl, G. (2009). Pleural tuberculosis in patients with early HIV infection is associated with increased TNF-alpha expression and necrosis in granulomas. *PLoS One, 4*(1), e4228.

Bhatt, K., & Salgame, P. (2007). Host innate immune response to Mycobacterium tuberculosis. *Journal of Clinical Immunology, 27*(4), 347–362.

Bodnar, K. A., Serbina, N. V., & Flynn, J. L. (2001). Fate of Mycobacterium tuberculosis within murine dendritic cells. *Infection and Immunity, 69*(2), 800–809.

Boisson-Dupuis, S., El Baghdadi, J., Parvaneh, N., Bousfiha, A., Bustamante, J., Feinberg, J., et al. (2011). IL-12Rbeta1 deficiency in two of fifty children with severe tuberculosis from Iran, Morocco, and Turkey. *PLoS One, 6*(4), e18524.

Bonecini-Almeida, M. G., Ho, J. L., Boechat, N., Huard, R. C., Chitale, S., Doo, H., et al. (2004). Down- modulation of lung immune responses by interleukin-10 and transforming growth factor beta (TGF-beta) and analysis of TGF-beta receptors I and II in active tuberculosis. *Infection and Immunity, 72*(5), 2628–2634.

Boselli, D., Losana, G., Bernabei, P., Bosisio, D., Drysdale, P., Kiessling, R., et al. (2007). IFN-gamma regulates Fas ligand expression in human CD4+ T lymphocytes and controls their antimycobacterial cytotoxic functions. *European Journal of Immunology, 37*(8), 2196–2204.

Bourigault, M. L., Vacher, R., Rose, S., Olleros, M. L., Janssens, J. P., Quesniaux, V. F., et al. (2013). Tumor necrosis factor neutralization combined with chemotherapy enhances Mycobacterium tuberculosis clearance and reduces lung pathology. *American Journal of Clinical and Experimental Immunology, 2*(1), 124–134.

Bowdish, D. M., Sakamoto, K., Kim, M. J., Kroos, M., Mukhopadhyay, S., Leifer, C. A., et al. (2009). MARCO, TLR2, and CD14 are required for macrophage cytokine responses to mycobacterial trehalose dimycolate and Mycobacterium tuberculosis. *PLoS Pathogens, 5*(6), e1000474.

Bulut, Y., Michelsen, K. S., Hayrapetian, L., Naiki, Y., Spallek, R., Singh, M., et al. (2005). Mycobacterium tuberculosis heat shock proteins use diverse toll-like receptor pathways to activate pro-inflammatory signals. *The Journal of Biological Chemistry, 280*(22), 20961–20967.

Cadena, A. M., Fortune, S. M., & Flynn, J. L. (2017). Heterogeneity in tuberculosis. *Nature Reviews. Immunology, 17*(11), 691–702.

Carmona, J., Cruz, A., Moreira-Teixeira, L., Sousa, C., Sousa, J., Osorio, N. S., et al. (2013). Mycobacterium tuberculosis strains are differentially recognized by TLRs with an impact on the immune response. *PLoS One, 8*(6), e67277.

Cassatella, M. A., Gasperini, S., Bovolenta, C., Calzetti, F., Vollebregt, M., Scapini, P., et al. (1999). Interleukin-10 (IL-10) selectively enhances CIS3/SOCS3 mRNA expression in human neutrophils: Evidence for an IL-10-induced pathway that is independent of STAT protein activation. *Blood, 94*(8), 2880–2889.

Chakravarty, S. D., Zhu, G., Tsai, M. C., Mohan, V. P., Marino, S., Kirschner, D. E., et al. (2008). Tumor necrosis factor blockade in chronic murine tuberculosis enhances granulomatous inflammation and disorganizes granulomas in the lungs. *Infection and Immunity, 76*(3), 916–926.

Chan, J., Mehta, S., Bharrhan, S., Chen, Y., Achkar, J. M., Casadevall, A., et al. (2014). The role of B cells and humoral immunity in Mycobacterium tuberculosis infection. *Seminars in Immunology, 26*(6), 588–600.

Chatterjee, S. B., Dey, S., Shi, W. Y., Thomas, K., & Hutchins, G. M. (1997). Accumulation of glycosphingolipids in human atherosclerotic plaque and unaffected aorta tissues. *Glycobiology, 7*(1), 57–65.

Collins, H. L., & Kaufmann, S. H. (2001). The many faces of host responses to tuberculosis. *Immunology, 103*(1), 1–9.

Condos, R., Rom, W. N., Liu, Y. M., & Schluger, N. W. (1998). Local immune responses correlate with presentation and outcome in tuberculosis. *American Journal of Respiratory and Critical Care Medicine, 157*(3 Pt 1), 729–735.

Cooper, A. M. (2009). Cell-mediated immune responses in tuberculosis. *Annual Review of Immunology, 27*, 393–422.

Cooper, A. M., Mayer-Barber, K. D., & Sher, A. (2011). Role of innate cytokines in mycobacterial infection. *Mucosal Immunology, 4*(3), 252–260.

Cruz, A., Fraga, A. G., Fountain, J. J., Rangel-Moreno, J., Torrado, E., Saraiva, M., et al. (2010). Pathological role of interleukin 17 in mice subjected to repeated BCG vaccination after infection with Mycobacterium tuberculosis. *The Journal of Experimental Medicine, 207*(8), 1609–1616.

Cun, X., Xie, J., Lin, S., Fu, N., Deng, S., Xie, Q., et al. (2015). Gene profile of soluble growth factors involved in angiogenesis, in an adipose-derived stromal cell/endothelial cell co-culture, 3D gel model. *Cell Proliferation, 48*(4), 405–412.

Dang, E. V., Barbi, J., Yang, H. Y., Jinasena, D., Yu, H., Zheng, Y., et al. (2011). Control of T(H)17/T(reg) balance by hypoxia-inducible factor 1. *Cell, 146*(5), 772–784.

Daniel, T. M., Oxtoby, M. J., Pinto, E., & Moreno, E. (1981). The immune spectrum in patients with pulmonary tuberculosis. *The American Review of Respiratory Disease, 123*(5), 556–559.

Daniel, J., Maamar, H., Deb, C., Sirakova, T. D., & Kolattukudy, P. E. (2011). Mycobacterium tuberculosis uses host triacylglycerol to accumulate lipid droplets and acquires a dormancy-like phenotype in lipid-loaded macrophages. *PLoS Pathogens, 7*(6), e1002093.

Datta, M., Via, L. E., Kamoun, W. S., Liu, C., Chen, W., Seano, G., et al. (2015). Anti-vascular endothelial growth factor treatment normalizes tuberculosis granuloma vasculature and improves small molecule delivery. *Proceedings of the National Academy of Sciences of the United States of America, 112*(6), 1827–1832.

Davis, J. M., & Ramakrishnan, L. (2009). The role of the granuloma in expansion and dissemination of early tuberculous infection. *Cell, 136*(1), 37–49.

de Valliere, S., Abate, G., Blazevic, A., Heuertz, R. M., & Hoft, D. F. (2005). Enhancement of innate and cell-mediated immunity by antimycobacterial antibodies. *Infection and Immunity, 73*(10), 6711–6720.

Desel, C., Dorhoi, A., Bandermann, S., Grode, L., Eisele, B., & Kaufmann, S. H. (2011). Recombinant BCG DeltaureC hly+ induces superior protection over parental BCG by stimulating a balanced combination of type 1 and type 17 cytokine responses. *The Journal of Infectious Diseases, 204*(10), 1573–1584.

Dhiman, R., Indramohan, M., Barnes, P. F., Nayak, R. C., Paidipally, P., Rao, L. V., et al. (2009). IL-22 produced by human NK cells inhibits growth of Mycobacterium tuberculosis by enhancing phagolysosomal fusion. *Journal of Immunology, 183*(10), 6639–6645.

Dhiman, R., Venkatasubramanian, S., Paidipally, P., Barnes, P. F., Tvinnereim, A., & Vankayalapati, R. (2014). Interleukin 22 inhibits intracellular growth of Mycobacterium tuberculosis by enhancing calgranulin a expression. *The Journal of Infectious Diseases, 209*(4), 578–587.

Divangahi, M., Mostowy, S., Coulombe, F., Kozak, R., Guillot, L., Veyrier, F., et al. (2008). NOD2-deficient mice have impaired resistance to Mycobacterium tuberculosis infection through defective innate and adaptive immunity. *Journal of Immunology, 181*(10), 7157–7165.

Domingo-Gonzalez, R., Prince, O., Cooper, A., & Khader, S. A. (2016). Cytokines and chemokines in Mycobacterium tuberculosis infection. *Microbiology Spectrum, 4*(5). https://doi.org/10.1128/microbiolspec.TBTB2-0018-2016.

du Preez, I., & Loots, D. T. (2013). New sputum metabolite markers implicating adaptations of the host to Mycobacterium tuberculosis, and vice versa. *Tuberculosis (Edinburgh, Scotland), 93*(3), 330–337.

Encinales, L., Zuniga, J., Granados-Montiel, J., Yunis, M., Granados, J., Almeciga, I., et al. (2010). Humoral immunity in tuberculin skin test anergy and its role in high-risk persons exposed to active tuberculosis. *Molecular Immunology, 47*(5), 1066–1073.

Fahey, T. J., 3rd, Tracey, K. J., Tekamp-Olson, P., Cousens, L. S., Jones, W. G., Shires, G. T., et al. (1992). Macrophage inflammatory protein 1 modulates macrophage function. *Journal of Immunology, 148*(9), 2764–2769.

Feng, L., Li, L., Liu, Y., Qiao, D., Li, Q., Fu, X., et al. (2011). B lymphocytes that migrate to tuberculous pleural fluid via the SDF-1/CXCR4 axis actively respond to antigens specific for Mycobacterium tuberculosis. *European Journal of Immunology, 41*(11), 3261–3269.

Fielding, C. A., McLoughlin, R. M., McLeod, L., Colmont, C. S., Najdovska, M., Grail, D., et al. (2008). IL-6 regulates neutrophil trafficking during acute inflammation via STAT3. *Journal of Immunology, 181*(3), 2189–2195.

Flynn, J. L., & Chan, J. (2005). What's good for the host is good for the bug. *Trends in Microbiology, 13*(3), 98–102.

Flynn, J. L., Chan, J., & Lin, P. L. (2011). Macrophages and control of granulomatous inflammation in tuberculosis. *Mucosal Immunology, 4*(3), 271–278.

Frieden, T. R., Sterling, T. R., Munsiff, S. S., Watt, C. J., & Dye, C. (2003). Tuberculosis. *Lancet, 362*(9387), 887–899.

Garner, B., Mellor, H. R., Butters, T. D., Dwek, R. A., & Platt, F. M. (2002). Modulation of THP-1 macrophage and cholesterol-loaded foam cell apolipoprotein E levels by glycosphingolipids. *Biochemical and Biophysical Research Communications, 290*(5), 1361–1367.

Geijtenbeek, T. B., Van Vliet, S. J., Koppel, E. A., Sanchez-Hernandez, M., Vandenbroucke-Grauls, C. M., Appelmelk, B., et al. (2003). Mycobacteria target DC-SIGN to suppress dendritic cell function. *The Journal of Experimental Medicine, 197*(1), 7–17.

Gopal, R., Rangel-Moreno, J., Slight, S., Lin, Y., Nawar, H. F., Fallert Junecko, B. A., et al. (2013). Interleukin-17-dependent CXCL13 mediates mucosal vaccine-induced immunity against tuberculosis. *Mucosal Immunology, 6*(5), 972–984.

Gordon, S. (2003). Alternative activation of macrophages. *Nature Reviews. Immunology, 3*(1), 23–35.

Guilliams, M., Bruhns, P., Saeys, Y., Hammad, H., & Lambrecht, B. N. (2014). The function of Fcgamma receptors in dendritic cells and macrophages. *Nature Reviews. Immunology, 14*(2), 94–108.

Hamasur, B., Haile, M., Pawlowski, A., Schroder, U., Kallenius, G., & Svenson, S. B. (2004). A mycobacterial lipoarabinomannan specific monoclonal antibody and its F(ab') fragment prolong survival of mice infected with Mycobacterium tuberculosis. *Clinical and Experimental Immunology, 138*(1), 30–38.

Harris, J., De Haro, S. A., Master, S. S., Keane, J., Roberts, E. A., Delgado, M., et al. (2007). T helper 2 cytokines inhibit autophagic control of intracellular Mycobacterium tuberculosis. *Immunity, 27*(3), 505–517.

Heitmann, L., Abad Dar, M., Schreiber, T., Erdmann, H., Behrends, J., McKenzie, A. N., et al. (2014). The IL-13/IL-4Ralpha axis is involved in tuberculosis-associated pathology. *The Journal of Pathology, 234*(3), 338–350.

Hemmi, H., Takeuchi, O., Kawai, T., Kaisho, T., Sato, S., Sanjo, H., et al. (2000). A toll-like receptor recognizes bacterial DNA. *Nature, 408*(6813), 740–745.

Hoheisel, G., Izbicki, G., Roth, M., Chan, C. H., Leung, J. C., Reichenberger, F., et al. (1998). Compartmentalization of pro-inflammatory cytokines in tuberculous pleurisy. *Respiratory Medicine, 92*(1), 14–17.

Hossain, M. M., & Norazmi, M. N. (2013). Pattern recognition receptors and cytokines in Mycobacterium tuberculosis infection--the double-edged sword? *BioMed Research International, 2013*, 179174.

Hsieh, C. H., Frink, M., Hsieh, Y. C., Kan, W. H., Hsu, J. T., Schwacha, M. G., et al. (2008). The role of MIP-1 alpha in the development of systemic inflammatory response and organ injury following trauma hemorrhage. *Journal of Immunology, 181*(4), 2806–2812.

Hussain, R., Ansari, A., Talat, N., Hasan, Z., & Dawood, G. (2011). CCL2/MCP-I genotype- phenotype relationship in latent tuberculosis infection. *PLoS One, 6*(10), e25803.

Huynh, K. K., Joshi, S. A., & Brown, E. J. (2011). A delicate dance: Host response to mycobacteria. *Current Opinion in Immunology, 23*(4), 464–472.

Jacobs, A. J., Mongkolsapaya, J., Screaton, G. R., McShane, H., & Wilkinson, R. J. (2016). Antibodies and tuberculosis. *Tuberculosis (Edinburgh, Scotland), 101*, 102–113.

Jones, L. L., & Vignali, D. A. (2011). Molecular interactions within the IL-6/IL-12 cytokine/receptor superfamily. *Immunologic Research, 51*(1), 5–14.

Joosten, S. A., van Meijgaarden, K. E., Del Nonno, F., Baiocchini, A., Petrone, L., Vanini, V., et al. (2016). Patients with tuberculosis have a dysfunctional circulating B-cell compartment, which normalizes following successful treatment. *PLoS Pathogens, 12*(6), e1005687.

Kaplan, G., Post, F. A., Moreira, A. L., Wainwright, H., Kreiswirth, B. N., Tanverdi, M., et al. (2003). Mycobacterium tuberculosis growth at the cavity surface: A microenvironment with failed immunity. *Infection and Immunity, 71*(12), 7099–7108.

Keane, J., Gershon, S., Wise, R. P., Mirabile-Levens, E., Kasznica, J., Schwieterman, W. D., et al. (2001). Tuberculosis associated with infliximab, a tumor necrosis factor alpha- neutralizing agent. *The New England Journal of Medicine, 345*(15), 1098–1104.

Khader, S. A., Partida-Sanchez, S., Bell, G., Jelley-Gibbs, D. M., Swain, S., Pearl, J. E., et al. (2006). Interleukin 12p40 is required for dendritic cell migration and T cell priming after Mycobacterium tuberculosis infection. *The Journal of Experimental Medicine, 203*(7), 1805–1815.

Khader, S. A., Bell, G. K., Pearl, J. E., Fountain, J. J., Rangel-Moreno, J., Cilley, G. E., et al. (2007). IL-23 and IL-17 in the establishment of protective pulmonary CD4+ T cell responses after vaccination and during Mycobacterium tuberculosis challenge. *Nature Immunology, 8*(4), 369–377.

Khader, S. A., Guglani, L., Rangel-Moreno, J., Gopal, R., Junecko, B. A., Fountain, J. J., et al. (2011). IL-23 is required for long-term control of Mycobacterium tuberculosis and B cell follicle formation in the infected lung. *Journal of Immunology, 187*(10), 5402–5407.

Kim, M. J., Wainwright, H. C., Locketz, M., Bekker, L. G., Walther, G. B., Dittrich, C., et al. (2010). Caseation of human tuberculosis granulomas correlates with elevated host lipid metabolism. *EMBO Molecular Medicine, 2*(7), 258–274.

Kinjo, Y., Kawakami, K., Uezu, K., Yara, S., Miyagi, K., Koguchi, Y., et al. (2002). Contribution of IL-18 to Th1 response and host defense against infection by Mycobacterium tuberculosis: A comparative study with IL-12p40. *Journal of Immunology, 169*(1), 323–329.

Kiran, D., Podell, B. K., Chambers, M., & Basaraba, R. J. (2016). Host-directed therapy targeting the Mycobacterium tuberculosis granuloma: A review. *Seminars in Immunopathology, 38*(2), 167–183.

Kohmo, S., Kijima, T., Mori, M., Minami, T., Namba, Y., Yano, Y., et al. (2012). CXCL12 as a biological marker for the diagnosis of tuberculous pleurisy. *Tuberculosis (Edinburgh, Scotland), 92*(3), 248–252.

Kolloli, A., & Subbian, S. (2017). Host-directed therapeutic strategies for tuberculosis. *Frontiers in Medicine (Lausanne), 4*, 171.

Koo, M. S., Manca, C., Yang, G., O'Brien, P., Sung, N., Tsenova, L., et al. (2011). Phosphodiesterase 4 inhibition reduces innate immunity and improves isoniazid clearance of Mycobacterium tuberculosis in the lungs of infected mice. *PLoS One, 6*(2), e17091.

Kozakiewicz, L., Phuah, J., Flynn, J., & Chan, J. (2013). The role of B cells and humoral immunity in Mycobacterium tuberculosis infection. *Advances in Experimental Medicine and Biology, 783*, 225–250.

Kramnik, I., & Beamer, G. (2016). Mouse models of human TB pathology: Roles in the analysis of necrosis and the development of host-directed therapies. *Seminars in Immunopathology, 38*(2), 221–237.

Krutzik, S. R., Ochoa, M. T., Sieling, P. A., Uematsu, S., Ng, Y. W., Legaspi, A., et al. (2003). Activation and regulation of toll-like receptors 2 and 1 in human leprosy. *Nature Medicine, 9*(5), 525–532.

Kumar, N. P., Gopinath, V., Sridhar, R., Hanna, L. E., Banurekha, V. V., Jawahar, M. S., et al. (2013). IL-10 dependent suppression of type 1, type 2 and type 17 cytokines in active pulmonary tuberculosis. *PLoS One, 8*(3), e59572.

Kumar, S. K., Singh, P., & Sinha, S. (2015). Naturally produced opsonizing antibodies restrict the survival of Mycobacterium tuberculosis in human macrophages by augmenting phagosome maturation. *Open Biology, 5*(12), 150171.

Kumar, N. P., Banurekha, V. V., Nair, D., & Babu, S. (2016). Circulating angiogenic factors as biomarkers of disease severity and bacterial burden in pulmonary tuberculosis. *PLoS One, 11*(1), e0146318.

Ladel, C. H., Blum, C., Dreher, A., Reifenberg, K., & Kaufmann, S. H. (1995). Protective role of gamma/delta T cells and alpha/beta T cells in tuberculosis. *European Journal of Immunology, 25*(10), 2877–2881.

Law, K., Weiden, M., Harkin, T., Tchou-Wong, K., Chi, C., & Rom, W. N. (1996). Increased release of interleukin-1 beta, interleukin-6, and tumor necrosis factor-alpha by bronchoalveolar cells lavaged from involved sites in pulmonary tuberculosis. *American Journal of Respiratory and Critical Care Medicine, 153*(2), 799–804.

Lin, P. L., & Flynn, J. L. (2010). Understanding latent tuberculosis: A moving target. *Journal of Immunology, 185*(1), 15–22.

Lin, P. L., Rodgers, M., Smith, L., Bigbee, M., Myers, A., Bigbee, C., et al. (2009). Quantitative comparison of active and latent tuberculosis in the cynomolgus macaque model. *Infection and Immunity, 77*(10), 4631–4642.

Lin, P. L., Rutledge, T., Green, A. M., Bigbee, M., Fuhrman, C., Klein, E., et al. (2012). CD4 T cell depletion exacerbates acute Mycobacterium tuberculosis while reactivation of latent infection is dependent on severity of tissue depletion in cynomolgus macaques. *AIDS Research and Human Retroviruses, 28*(12), 1693–1702.

Lindenstrom, T., Woodworth, J., Dietrich, J., Aagaard, C., Andersen, P., & Agger, E. M. (2012). Vaccine-induced th17 cells are maintained long-term postvaccination as a distinct and phenotypically stable memory subset. *Infection and Immunity, 80*(10), 3533–3544.

Lingnau, M., Hoflich, C., Volk, H. D., Sabat, R., & Docke, W. D. (2007). Interleukin-10 enhances the CD14-dependent phagocytosis of bacteria and apoptotic cells by human monocytes. *Human Immunology, 68*(9), 730–738.

Liu, P. T., Schenk, M., Walker, V. P., Dempsey, P. W., Kanchanapoomi, M., Wheelwright, M., et al. (2009). Convergence of IL-1beta and VDR activation pathways in human TLR2/1-induced antimicrobial responses. *PLoS One, 4*(6), e5810.

Lockhart, E., Green, A. M., & Flynn, J. L. (2006). IL-17 production is dominated by gammadelta T cells rather than CD4 T cells during Mycobacterium tuberculosis infection. *Journal of Immunology, 177*(7), 4662–4669.

Lugo-Villarino, G., Hudrisier, D., Benard, A., & Neyrolles, O. (2012). Emerging trends in the formation and function of tuberculosis granulomas. *Frontiers in Immunology, 3*, 405.

Maglione, P. J., Xu, J., & Chan, J. (2007). B cells moderate inflammatory progression and enhance bacterial containment upon pulmonary challenge with Mycobacterium tuberculosis. *Journal of Immunology, 178*(11), 7222–7234.

Maglione, P. J., Xu, J., Casadevall, A., & Chan, J. (2008). Fc gamma receptors regulate immune activation and susceptibility during Mycobacterium tuberculosis infection. *Journal of Immunology, 180*(5), 3329–3338.

Marino, S., El-Kebir, M., & Kirschner, D. (2011). A hybrid multi-compartment model of granuloma formation and T cell priming in tuberculosis. *Journal of Theoretical Biology, 280*(1), 50–62.

Master, S. S., Rampini, S. K., Davis, A. S., Keller, C., Ehlers, S., Springer, B., et al. (2008). Mycobacterium tuberculosis prevents inflammasome activation. *Cell Host & Microbe, 3*(4), 224–232.

Matthews, K., Wilkinson, K. A., Kalsdorf, B., Roberts, T., Diacon, A., Walzl, G., et al. (2011). Predominance of interleukin-22 over interleukin-17 at the site of disease in human tuberculosis. *Tuberculosis (Edinburgh, Scotland), 91*(6), 587–593.

Mattila, J. T., Ojo, O. O., Kepka-Lenhart, D., Marino, S., Kim, J. H., Eum, S. Y., et al. (2013). Microenvironments in tuberculous granulomas are delineated by distinct populations of macrophage subsets and expression of nitric oxide synthase and arginase isoforms. *Journal of Immunology, 191*(2), 773–784.

Mazzarella, G., Bianco, A., Perna, F., D'Auria, D., Grella, E., Moscariello, E., et al. (2003). T lymphocyte phenotypic profile in lung segments affected by cavitary and non-cavitary tuberculosis. *Clinical and Experimental Immunology, 132*(2), 283–288.

McAleer, J. P., & Kolls, J. K. (2014). Directing traffic: IL-17 and IL-22 coordinate pulmonary immune defense. *Immunological Reviews, 260*(1), 129–144.

Moore, K. W., de Waal Malefyt, R., Coffman, R. L., & O'Garra, A. (2001). Interleukin-10 and the interleukin-10 receptor. *Annual Review of Immunology, 19*, 683–765.

Moser, B., & Loetscher, P. (2001). Lymphocyte traffic control by chemokines. *Nature Immunology, 2*(2), 123–128.

Nandi, B., & Behar, S. M. (2011). Regulation of neutrophils by interferon-gamma limits lung inflammation during tuberculosis infection. *The Journal of Experimental Medicine, 208*(11), 2251–2262.

Nigou, J., Zelle-Rieser, C., Gilleron, M., Thurnher, M., & Puzo, G. (2001). Mannosylated lipoarabinomannans inhibit IL-12 production by human dendritic cells: Evidence for a negative signal delivered through the mannose receptor. *Journal of Immunology, 166*(12), 7477–7485.

O'Garra, A., Redford, P. S., McNab, F. W., Bloom, C. I., Wilkinson, R. J., & Berry, M. P. (2013). The immune response in tuberculosis. *Annual Review of Immunology, 31*, 475–527.

O'Kane, C. M., Boyle, J. J., Horncastle, D. E., Elkington, P. T., & Friedland, J. S. (2007). Monocyte-dependent fibroblast CXCL8 secretion occurs in tuberculosis and limits survival of mycobacteria within macrophages. *Journal of Immunology, 178*(6), 3767–3776.

O'Leary, S., O'Sullivan, M. P., & Keane, J. (2011). IL-10 blocks phagosome maturation in mycobacterium tuberculosis-infected human macrophages. *American Journal of Respiratory Cell and Molecular Biology, 45*(1), 172–180.

Oehlers, S. H., Cronan, M. R., Scott, N. R., Thomas, M. I., Okuda, K. S., Walton, E. M., et al. (2015). Interception of host angiogenic signalling limits mycobacterial growth. *Nature, 517*(7536), 612–615.

Okamoto Yoshida, Y., Umemura, M., Yahagi, A., O'Brien, R. L., Ikuta, K., Kishihara, K., et al. (2010). Essential role of IL-17A in the formation of a mycobacterial infection-induced granuloma in the lung. *Journal of Immunology, 184*(8), 4414–4422.

Olivares, N., Puig, A., Aguilar, D., Moya, A., Cadiz, A., Otero, O., et al. (2009). Prophylactic effect of administration of human gamma globulins in a mouse model of tuberculosis. *Tuberculosis (Edinburgh, Scotland), 89*(3), 218–220.

Ordway, D., Henao-Tamayo, M., Harton, M., Palanisamy, G., Troudt, J., Shanley, C., et al. (2007). The hypervirulent Mycobacterium tuberculosis strain HN878 induces a potent TH1 response followed by rapid down-regulation. *Journal of Immunology, 179*(1), 522–531.

Osherov, N., & Ben-Ami, R. (2016). Modulation of host angiogenesis as a microbial survival strategy and therapeutic target. *PLoS Pathogens, 12*(4), e1005479.

Pahari, S., Kaur, G., Aqdas, M., Negi, S., Chatterjee, D., Bashir, H., et al. (2017). Bolstering immunity through pattern recognition receptors: A unique approach to control tuberculosis. *Frontiers in Immunology, 8*, 906.

Palsson-McDermott, E. M., Curtis, A. M., Goel, G., Lauterbach, M. A., Sheedy, F. J., Gleeson, L. E., et al. (2015). Pyruvate kinase M2 regulates Hif-1alpha activity and IL-1beta induction and is a critical determinant of the Warburg effect in LPS-activated macrophages. *Cell Metabolism, 21*(1), 65–80.

Pandey, A. K., & Sassetti, C. M. (2008). Mycobacterial persistence requires the utilization of host cholesterol. *Proceedings of the National Academy of Sciences of the United States of America, 105*(11), 4376–4380.

Pandey, A. K., Yang, Y., Jiang, Z., Fortune, S. M., Coulombe, F., Behr, M. A., et al. (2009). NOD2, RIP2 and IRF5 play a critical role in the type I interferon response to Mycobacterium tuberculosis. *PLoS Pathogens, 5*(7), e1000500.

Philips, J. A., & Ernst, J. D. (2012). Tuberculosis pathogenesis and immunity. *Annual Review of Pathology, 7*, 353–384.

Quesniaux, V., Fremond, C., Jacobs, M., Parida, S., Nicolle, D., Yeremeev, V., et al. (2004). Toll-like receptor pathways in the immune responses to mycobacteria. *Microbes and Infection, 6*(10), 946–959.

Rajaram, M. V. S., Arnett, E., Azad, A. K., Guirado, E., Ni, B., Gerberick, A. D., et al. (2017). M. tuberculosis-initiated human mannose receptor signaling regulates macrophage recognition and vesicle trafficking by FcRgamma-chain, Grb2, and SHP-1. *Cell Reports, 21*(1), 126–140.

Reiling, N., Holscher, C., Fehrenbach, A., Kroger, S., Kirschning, C. J., Goyert, S., et al. (2002). Cutting edge: Toll-like receptor (TLR)2- and TLR4-mediated pathogen recognition in resistance to airborne infection with Mycobacterium tuberculosis. *Journal of Immunology, 169*(7), 3480–3484.

Rodrigo, T., Cayla, J. A., Garcia de Olalla, P., Galdos-Tanguis, H., Jansa, J. M., Miranda, P., et al. (1997). Characteristics of tuberculosis patients who generate secondary cases. *The International Journal of Tuberculosis and Lung Disease, 1*(4), 352–357.

Russell, D. G., Cardona, P. J., Kim, M. J., Allain, S., & Altare, F. (2009a). Foamy macrophages and the progression of the human tuberculosis granuloma. *Nature Immunology, 10*(9), 943–948.

Russell, D. G., Vanderven, B. C., Glennie, S., Mwandumba, H., & Heyderman, R. S. (2009b). The macrophage marches on its phagosome: Dynamic assays of phagosome function. *Nature Reviews. Immunology, 9*(8), 594–600.

Sakai, H., Okafuji, I., Nishikomori, R., Abe, J., Izawa, K., Kambe, N., et al. (2010). The CD40-CD40L axis and IFN-gamma play critical roles in Langhans giant cell formation. *International Immunology, 24*(1), 5–15.

Saukkonen, J. J., Bazydlo, B., Thomas, M., Strieter, R. M., Keane, J., & Kornfeld, H. (2002). Beta-chemokines are induced by Mycobacterium tuberculosis and inhibit its growth. *Infection and Immunity, 70*(4), 1684–1693.

Schlesinger, L. S., Hull, S. R., & Kaufman, T. M. (1994). Binding of the terminal mannosyl units of lipoarabinomannan from a virulent strain of Mycobacterium tuberculosis to human macrophages. *Journal of Immunology, 152*(8), 4070–4079.

Seiler, P., Aichele, P., Bandermann, S., Hauser, A. E., Lu, B., Gerard, N. P., et al. (2003). Early granuloma formation after aerosol Mycobacterium tuberculosis infection is regulated by neutrophils via CXCR3-signaling chemokines. *European Journal of Immunology, 33*(10), 2676–2686.

Semenza, G. L. (2010). HIF-1: upstream and downstream of cancer metabolism. *Current Opinion in Genetics and Development, 20*(1), 51–56.

Shalekoff, S., & Tiemessen, C. T. (2003). Circulating levels of stromal cell-derived factor 1alpha and interleukin 7 in HIV type 1 infection and pulmonary tuberculosis are reciprocally related to CXCR4 expression on peripheral blood leukocytes. *AIDS Research and Human Retroviruses, 19*(6), 461–468.

Shi, L., Eugenin, E. A., & Subbian, S. (2016). Immunometabolism in tuberculosis. *Frontiers in Immunology, 7*, 150.

Siveke, J. T., & Hamann, A. (1998). T helper 1 and T helper 2 cells respond differentially to chemokines. *Journal of Immunology, 160*(2), 550–554.

Stegelmann, F., Bastian, M., Swoboda, K., Bhat, R., Kiessler, V., Krensky, A. M., et al. (2005). Coordinate expression of CC chemokine ligand 5, granulysin, and perforin in CD8+ T cells provides a host defense mechanism against Mycobacterium tuberculosis. *Journal of Immunology, 175*(11), 7474–7483.

Strzelak, A., Komorowska-Piotrowska, A., & Ziolkowski, J. (2012). [CXCL10/IP-10 as a new biomarker for Mycobacterium tuberculosis infection]. *Polski Merkuriusz Lekarski, 33*(198), 342–345.

Subbian, S., Tsenova, L., Yang, G., O'Brien, P., Parsons, S., Peixoto, B., et al. (2011). Chronic pulmonary cavitary tuberculosis in rabbits: A failed host immune response. *Open Biology, 1*(4), 110016.

Suwara, M. I., Green, N. J., Borthwick, L. A., Mann, J., Mayer-Barber, K. D., Barron, L., et al. (2014). IL-1alpha released from damaged epithelial cells is sufficient and essential to trigger inflammatory responses in human lung fibroblasts. *Mucosal Immunology, 7*(3), 684–693.

Tabarsi, P., Marjani, M., Mansouri, N., Farnia, P., Boisson-Dupuis, S., Bustamante, J., et al. (2011). Lethal tuberculosis in a previously healthy adult with IL-12 receptor deficiency. *Journal of Clinical Immunology, 31*(4), 537–539.

Tan, S., & Russell, D. G. (2015). Trans-species communication in the Mycobacterium tuberculosis-infected macrophage. *Immunological Reviews, 264*(1), 233–248.

Toossi, Z., & Ellner, J. J. (1998). The role of TGF beta in the pathogenesis of human tuberculosis. *Clinical Immunology and Immunopathology, 87*(2), 107–114.

Toossi, Z., Gogate, P., Shiratsuchi, H., Young, T., & Ellner, J. J. (1995). Enhanced production of TGF-beta by blood monocytes from patients with active tuberculosis and presence of TGF-beta in tuberculous granulomatous lung lesions. *Journal of Immunology, 154*(1), 465–473.

Tsenova, L., O'Brien, P., Holloway, J., Peixoto, B., Soteropoulos, P., Fallows, D., et al. (2014). Etanercept exacerbates inflammation and pathology in a rabbit model of active pulmonary tuberculosis. *Journal of Interferon & Cytokine Research, 34*(9), 716–726.

Uehira, K., Amakawa, R., Ito, T., Tajima, K., Naitoh, S., Ozaki, Y., et al. (2002). Dendritic cells are decreased in blood and accumulated in granuloma in tuberculosis. *Clinical Immunology, 105*(3), 296–303.

Ulrichs, T., Kosmiadi, G. A., Jörg, S., Pradl, L., Titukhina, M., Mishenko, V., et al. (2005). Differential organization of the local immune response in patients with active cavitary tuberculosis or with nonprogressive tuberculoma. *The Journal of Infectious Diseases, 192*(1), 89–97.

Verway, M., Bouttier, M., Wang, T. T., Carrier, M., Calderon, M., An, B. S., et al. (2013). Vitamin D induces interleukin-1beta expression: Paracrine macrophage epithelial signaling controls M. tuberculosis infection. *PLoS Pathogens, 9*(6), e1003407.

Vesosky, B., Rottinghaus, E. K., Stromberg, P., Turner, J., & Beamer, G. (2010). CCL5 participates in early protection against Mycobacterium tuberculosis. *Journal of Leukocyte Biology, 87*(6), 1153–1165.

Wallis, R. S., Kyambadde, P., Johnson, J. L., Horter, L., Kittle, R., Pohle, M., et al. (2004). A study of the safety, immunology, virology, and microbiology of adjunctive etanercept in HIV-1-associated tuberculosis. *AIDS, 18*(2), 257–264.

Welsh, K. J., Risin, S. A., Actor, J. K., & Hunter, R. L. (2011). Immunopathology of postprimary tuberculosis: Increased T-regulatory cells and DEC-205-positive foamy macrophages in cavitary lesions. *Clinical & Developmental Immunology, 2011*, 307631.

WHO. (2017). *Global tuberculosis report*. Geneva: World Health Organization.

Wieland, C. W., van der Windt, G. J., Wiersinga, W. J., Florquin, S., & van der Poll, T. (2008). CD14 contributes to pulmonary inflammation and mortality during murine tuberculosis. *Immunology, 125*(2), 272–279.

Wozniak, T. M., Ryan, A. A., & Britton, W. J. (2006). Interleukin-23 restores immunity to Mycobacterium tuberculosis infection in IL-12p40-deficient mice and is not required for the development of IL-17-secreting T cell responses. *Journal of Immunology, 177*(12), 8684–8692.

Zhang, Y., Lathigra, R., Garbe, T., Catty, D., & Young, D. (1991). Genetic analysis of superoxide dismutase, the 23 kilodalton antigen of Mycobacterium tuberculosis. *Molecular Microbiology, 5*(2), 381–391.

Zhang, Z., Kaptanoglu, L., Tang, Y., Ivancic, D., Rao, S. M., Luster, A., et al. (2004). IP-10-induced recruitment of CXCR3 host T cells is required for small bowel allograft rejection. *Gastroenterology, 126*(3), 809–818.

Zumla, A., Raviglione, M., Hafner, R., & von Reyn, C. F. (2013). Tuberculosis. *The New England Journal of Medicine, 368*(8), 745–755.

Animal Models of Tuberculosis

Pooja Singh, Afsal Kolloli, and Selvakumar Subbian

Introduction

Tuberculosis (TB), an ancient disease that has evolved with humans for more than 4,000 years, still continues as a leading infectious disease of mankind across the world. Tuberculosis is caused by exposure to the bacteria of *Mycobacterium tuberculosis* (Mtb) complex, one of the most successful pathogen and a leading cause of morbidity and mortality in humans worldwide. In 2016, there were about 10.4 million new TB cases and 1.7 million deaths reported globally. Following exposure to aerosols containing Mtb, about 5% of individuals develop symptomatic pulmonary TB (primary TB); however, more than 90% of individuals exposed to Mtb (about a third of world population) are believed to be latently infected (latent tuberculosis infection, LTBI), without any clinical symptoms of active disease. However, these LTBI cases can develop symptomatic, progressive TB disease (reactivation TB or post-primary TB) upon host immune-compromising conditions; thus, LTBI serves as potential reservoir for future active TB cases. Furthermore, emergence of drug-resistant strains of Mtb and coexistence of TB with HIV and/or other chronic diseases further increases the burden on the death toll and poses significant health threat (WHO 2017). Our inability to control TB effectively lies on the issues associated with diagnosis, vaccination and treatment of the disease. In TB endemic countries, traditional microscopic sputum examination and tuberculin skin test are used routinely to diagnose TB; these methodologies have poor sensitivity and specificity, respectively (Tsara et al. 2009). In addition, advanced molecular diagnostic methods are not cost effective for TB endemic countries and are inconsistent in their diagnostic potential. These factors contribute to noncompliance of individuals

P. Singh · A. Kolloli · S. Subbian (✉)
Public Health Research Institute, New Jersey Medical School at Rutgers Biomedical and Health Sciences, Rutgers University, Newark, NJ, USA
e-mail: subbiase@njms.rutgers.edu

© Springer Nature Switzerland AG 2018
V. Venketaraman (ed.), *Understanding the Host Immune Response Against Mycobacterium tuberculosis Infection*, https://doi.org/10.1007/978-3-319-97367-8_4

suspected of active TB from diagnosis and enrollment for the treatment (Tsara et al. 2009). Therefore, improvised and cost-effective diagnostic modalities are required for efficient control of TB in endemic countries that contribute to about 80% of TB cases worldwide. Similarly, there is no effective vaccine available to prevent TB epidemic across various populations. The currently-prescribed vaccine against TB, BCG (bacille Calmette Guérin), derived from *Mycobacterium bovis*, has a highly variable (0–80%) protective efficacy in preventing childhood TB and does not protect against TB in adult population (Orme 2011). Hence, new and/or improved TB vaccine(s), capable of protecting children, adults, as well as immunocompromised people, is urgently needed. Finally, the current treatment regimen for drug-sensitive TB, namely DOTS (Directly Observed Treatment, Short course) is comprised of four antibiotics (isoniazid, rifampicin, ethambutol, and pyrazinamide) administered for 6 months. Due to longer duration of therapy and toxicity of the drugs, poor patient compliance has been reported for this treatment strategy. Taken together, there is an urgent need for future research to bring novel, innovative, and improved approaches in diagnosis, vaccine, and drug development for better management of global TB situation. In this context, various animal models of TB play pivotal role, such as to better understand the host-pathogen interactions during Mtb infection/ disease and to test new as well as improved drugs and vaccines (Fig. 1). In this

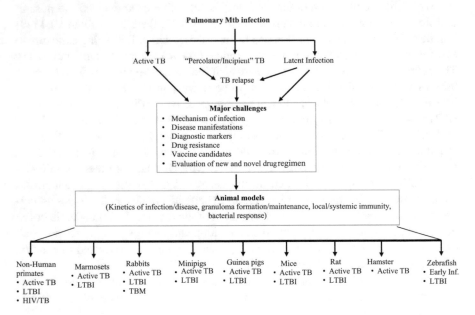

Fig. 1 Stages of Mtb infection/disease and the role of various animal models. Tuberculosis in humans encompasses active disease, latent TB infection, and relapse of infection/disease. Major challenges in TB study involve understanding the course of Mtb infection and the mechanisms to reduce bacterial burden and disease pathology. Animal models are the most effective and promising way to investigate these phenomena and to understand the role of host immune response toward Mtb infection. TB: tuberculosis; LTBI: latent TB; TBM: TB meningitis; HIV/TB: co-infection with HIV and TB

chapter, we discuss the salient features of various animal models of Mtb infection and their implications in TB research.

Overview of *Mycobacterium tuberculosis* Infection in Model Animals

Animal models serve as an excellent tool to study the course of Mtb infection (including acute/chronic active TB, LTBI, and reactivation), to understand the pathological manifestations of infection/disease, and to decipher the host and pathogen determinant(s) that are vital for pathogenesis. Knowledge gained from such studies can aid in developing more effective intervention strategies to combat TB in humans. Several animal models, ranging from zebrafish to nonhuman primates, have been explored to determine their resemblance of biological manifestations during Mtb infection/disease with corresponding human conditions; these model animals have been used successfully to various extents in TB research (Gupta and Katoch 2005). Each of these animal models, mainly of pulmonary Mtb infection/disease, mimic several clinical and pathological features seen in human TB patients, including pneumonia, various types of granulomas, and other features of disease (Fig. 1). Moreover, many animal models show more or less similar immune responses to Mtb infection, such as cytokine/chemokine production and cell-mediated immunity (Zhan et al. 2017). Importantly, each animal model of TB has its own advantages and limitations in reciprocating the infection/disease features and studying various aspects of human TB.

The ability of pathogenic Mtb to grow intracellularly and to cause disease in the infected host depends on several factors: (a) The virulence and fitness of Mtb, which is contributed by several secreted proteins and constituents of the bacterial cell wall structure. For example, mutant Mtb strains lacking ESAT-6, an early secreting antigen, are avirulent and do not cause effective infection in the host; similarly, variation in glycolipids influences the cytokine production and other effector functions of phagocytic cells. (b) The amount of infectious inoculum, which is associated with the severity of infection/disease caused by a particular Mtb strain. In general, a higher Mtb inoculum often results in severe infection and faster disease progression in many animal models of TB. (c) The genetic makeup of host. For example, studies have reported that outbred rabbits show different level of susceptibility to Mtb and *M. bovis* infection and that different strains of mice show varying levels of resistance to Mtb infection (Gupta and Katoch 2005). While all these animal models have been successful in providing insight into the progression of initial infection to chronic TB disease, differences in immune response to Mtb between different animal species make it challenging to relate the course of infection in humans (Table 1).

Table 1 Comparison of various animal models used in tuberculosis research

Animal models	Advantages	Disadvantages	Applications
Nonhuman primate	Physiological, anatomical, and genetic resemblance with human Granulomas with necrosis and cavitation Latent TB infection and co-infection with SIV Immunological reagents available	Difficult to handle Expensive Technical expertise Ethical issues	Immunological/host response to varying doses of TB infection Drug evaluation Vaccine candidates Treatment regimen
Marmoset	Physiological, anatomical, and genetic resemblance with human Granulomas with necrosis and cavitation Smaller size than NHP Easy to handle	Limited data available for Mtb infection Moderate level of immunological reagents availability Relatively more susceptible to Mtb infection Expensive Technical expertise	Host response to varying dose of infection Drug evaluation Preclinical studies
Rabbit	Granulomas with necrosis and cavitation Ease of handling Develops latency and reactivation spontaneously TB meningitis model	Limited availability of immunological reagents, Technical expertise	Cavitation TB meningitis model Vaccine testing Preclinical model for anti- TB drugs Host-directed therapies
Guinea pig/ hamster	Granulomas with necrosis Ease of handling	Latency not defined Relatively more susceptible to Mtb infection Limited availability of immunological reagents	Pathophysiology of TB Drug evaluation Vaccine efficacy
Minipig	Granulomas with necrosis Pediatric TB model	Expensive Limited immunological tools Difficult to handle Technical expertise Relatively more susceptible to Mtb infection	Immune response Mtb virulence testing Evaluating anti-TB drugs
Mouse/rat	Small size Easy to handle Inexpensive Availability of genetic variants Availability of immunological tools	Lacks granulomas with caseating necrosis or cavities True latency and reactivation not established	Mechanisms of immunological response Evaluation of drugs and vaccine candidates Gene expression and influence of disease progression Evaluation of Mtb and its components on granuloma formation
Zebrafish	Ease of breeding/handling Whole animal imaging Early stage granulomas	Lack lung structure and lymphocytes Lacks true granulomas with caseating necrosis and cavities, latency and reactivation not established	Role of innate immunity in granuloma formation Evaluation of Mtb and its components on granuloma formation Drug screening

Nonhuman Primates

Among various animal models of TB, nonhuman primates (NHP), such as macaques, are superior and provide excellent cellular and immunological insights about human pulmonary TB (Pena and Ho 2015). The NHPs are considered as the closest model animal to humans, and they have remarkable similarity in anatomical and pathological presentation of disease and immune response to Mtb infection (Carlsson et al. 2010). The use of NHP as a model for human Mtb infection dates back to 1960s when it was used for drug efficacy testing (Schmidt 1966). After which it was used to establish the role of BCG vaccination in protection against TB by several investigators. Between 1960s and 1970s was the "Golden age" of TB research, due to the extensive use of rhesus macaques that validated the role of BCG vaccination in establishing a protective immunity against pulmonary TB. Similar to humans, Mtb-infected NHPs display various outcomes of infection and disease events, such as latent TB, acute and active disease, as well as "percolator" and "insipient" forms of TB (Schmidt 1966; Capuano et al. 2003; Flynn 2006). In addition, macaque models also show similarity with human counterpart in their response to multiple drug treatment for TB and variable efficacy of BCG vaccination (Darrah et al. 2014; Larsen et al. 2009). Furthermore, macaque models have been used to study latent TB. Many immunological reagents available commercially for humans have been shown to be functional in this model, expanding the use of NHP in research addressing intricate and unique questions related to human TB (Flynn 2006).

The commonly used NHP models in TB research are the cynomolgus macaques (*Macaca fascicularis*) (CM), also known as long-tailed macaques and are native to Southeast Asia, and the Rhesus macaques (*Macaca mulatta*) (RM) native to Asia (Table 2). Although both RM and CM are very close to each other in many

Table 2 Various nonhuman primate models used in tuberculosis studies

Nonhuman primates	Agent of infection	Route of infection	Reference studies
Rhesus macaques (*Macaca mulatta*)	*Mtb* Erdman *M. Bovis* BCG *Mtb* CDC1551 *Mtb* H37Rv	Intravenous Intra-tracheal Aerosol	Shen et al. (2001); Janicki et al. (1973); Langermans et al. (2001); Darrah et al. (2014); Kaushal et al. (2015); Mothe et al. (2015); Phillips et al. (2017)
Cynomolgus macaque (*Macaca fascicularis*)	*Mtb* Erdman	Intra-tracheal	Lin et al. (2006, 2010); Diedrich et al. (2010); Maiello et al. (2018)
Marmosets (*Callithrix jacchus*)	*Mtb* Beijing strain *Mtb* CDC1551 *M. africanum* N0091	Aerosol	Via et al. (2013, 2015)

physiological and genetic features, some differences have been reported, mainly in their response to BCG vaccination (Langermans et al. 2001). Following Mtb infection, both RM and CM models develop all clinical forms of TB seen in human patients. These animals can be challenged with Mtb via different routes including, aerosol exposure and intra-bronchial or intra-tracheal instillation (Pena and Ho 2015). Although the route of infection influences distribution of disease in the lung, it does not significantly affect the overall pathological outcome of infection (Sibley et al. 2016). Development of TB in macaques can be diagnosed by TST, interferon gamma release assay (IGRA), chest X-ray, and sputum and/or culture positivity for Mtb (Vervenne et al. 2004). A typical representation of lung pathology in human TB, comprised of caseous granuloma, calcified regions, fibrous, pulmonary cavities or disseminated lesions, can also be observed in these macaque models of pulmonary TB. One of the pathological hallmarks of TB in human is the formation of granuloma, an organized cellular structure that is comprised of various types of immune cells surrounding infected phagocytes. Pulmonary granulomas of NHP model of TB share several similarities in their histopathological features and clinical manifestations of disease with human disease. Similar to humans, macaques develop heterogeneous granulomas following pulmonary Mtb infection, including fibro-calcific, non-necrotic and necrotic, and caseous, which can further progress to form cavities (Flynn et al. 2015; Mattila et al. 2013). In a CM model of Mtb infection, it has been shown that the macrophages with anti-inflammatory markers, such as arginase-1, are localized to the outer region of granuloma, whereas macrophages in the inner region of granuloma predominantly expressed pro-inflammatory markers, such as inducible nitric oxide synthase (Mattila et al. 2013). In addition, TNF-α neutralization in Mtb-infected macaques has been shown to cause reactivation and dissemination of Mtb and develop disease pathology, which underlines the role of TNF-α in the maintenance of granuloma integrity (Lin et al. 2010). Macaque model has also been used to study metabolic activities of immune cells as well as pathological transformation of the granuloma over time that can be imaged by PET/CT scanning coupled with FDG-labeling. Application of these technologies has helped to understand the correlation between granuloma integrity and disease progression in the NHP models (Lin et al. 2013). A recent PET/CT imaging study reported that inflammation following Mtb infection, marked by increased production of IL-2, IL-10, and IL-17 in the lung granulomas, contributes to reactivation of LTBI in CM (Wong et al. 2010). This model of Mtb infection also revealed that lymph nodes retain the bacteria after short-term anti-TB drug treatment; this Mtb population plays a potent role in disease reactivation as well as in disseminating the bacteria (Lin et al. 2012), thus suggesting that lymph nodes can act as a reservoir for infecting Mtb.

Macaque model of Mtb infection has been extensively used to investigate key host cell signaling mechanism during infection. Transcriptomic study of Mtb-infected lungs of NHP revealed the activation of pro-inflammatory signaling pathways, induced by cytokines such as TNF-α, IFN-γ, and chemokines, during early stages of Mtb infection. As the infection progresses, the immune cells in the lung granulomas undergo reprogramming to suppress the exacerbated inflammatory response (Mehra et al. 2010). Macaque model of active TB revealed that lung granulomas can undergo significant changes in structure and function at different stages of disease. Accordingly, an increased frequency of CD4+ and CD8+ cells were observed during active TB, whereas higher frequency of regulatory T cells (Tregs) was noted when LTBI ensues (Lin et al. 2009). These studies also suggest that a higher frequency of CD4+ Tregs in the blood as well as in the airways might have a role in the control of inflammation in animals with LTBI (Green et al. 2013).

Macaque model of vaccination followed by Mtb challenge is a standard procedure and has successfully been implicated in the evaluation of new and improved vaccines against TB, before conducting clinical trials in human population. Both the RM and CM models of TB have been used as potential tool to evaluate the efficacy of BCG-based and non-BCG derived vaccines and also to determine the Mtb infectious dosage as well as impact of route of inoculation on the outcome of infection. The CM are more resistant to low-dose Mtb infection and exhibit more effective protection to infection following BCG vaccination, compared to the RM, which are more susceptible to disease progression with high bacterial burden in lungs and extrapulmonary tissues. Various routes of BCG vaccination (i.e., intravenous, aerosol, or intra-cutaneous) were also tested in RM, and it was observed that aerosol vaccinated animals demonstrated no serological changes throughout the study time points, indicating no or poor onset protective immunity by this route. In contrast, positive anti-Mtb antibody reactivity was detected after 4 weeks of Mtb challenge in monkeys immunized with BCG intradermally; similar response was also noted at 8 weeks post infection in intravenously vaccinated animals, compared to 8–12 weeks in the unvaccinated group of challenged monkeys (Janicki et al. 1973). However, skin test with purified protein derivate of tuberculin (TST) was positive for all the groups of RM within 4 weeks of Mtb infection. The outcomes of this study showed variation in serological response after vaccination with BCG by different routes, which was attributed to the difference in immunological specificity and sensitivity of the host. Thus, skin reactivity was demonstrated as an early Mtb infection determinant over immunoglobulins A, G, and M (Janicki et al. 1973). These findings also suggest that RM model is more suitable to study acute and active TB, although CM model has been reported to be a better choice to study chronic TB and LTBI (Sharpe et al. 2009, 2016). Rhesus macaques were also tested for their similarity in producing immunodominant antigens during Mtb infection in humans. A recent study found that 54 immunodominant CD4+ T cell epitopes, including *Rv3875* (ESAT-6) and *Rv3874* (CFP10), were commonly expressed between human TB cases and Mtb-infected RM. This suggested the presence of several common MHC class II epitopes in human and macaques, thus justifying that vaccine candidate can be effectively screened in this model (Mothe et al. 2015).

Studies conducted in the RM model of pulmonary TB unveiled that a recombinant BCG (rBCG) vaccine (AFRO-1) enhances IFN-γ response and induces antigen-specific T cell proliferation (Rahman et al. 2009; Magalhaes et al. 2008). Similarly, prior vaccination of RM with BCG boosted by modified vaccinia virus Ankara-expressing antigen 85A (MVA.85A) and attenuated Mtb with a disrupted phoP gene induced IFN-γ response and provided significant protection against Mtb infection

(Verreck et al. 2009). Another study reported that the magnetic resonance imaging (MRI) is a better and more reliable readout to evaluate the efficacy of BCG-MVA.85 vaccine in RM model. The data from MRI readouts exhibit a significant correlation between Mtb burden in the granulomas and the immunological response in the lung (Luciw et al. 2011; Sharpe et al. 2010). In a CM model of TB, efficacy of a 72f rBCG vaccine (rBCG harboring 72f fusion gene) and DNA vaccine combination expressing mycobacterial heat shock protein 65 (Hsp65) and interleukin-12 (IL-12) (HSP65 + IL12) were evaluated. This study demonstrated that 72f rBCG as well as DNA-combination vaccines provided a better protection, compared to vaccination with BCG alone (Kita et al. 2013; Okada 2006). Similarly, boosting of BCG vaccine with a multistage H56 (H56/IC31) vaccine was shown to reduce the lung pathology and prevent the disease reactivation and dissemination even after TNF-α neutralization treatment in the CM model of Mtb infection (Lin et al. 2012).

The macaque model has also been used to evaluate the potency of different vaccine candidates, other than BCG or its derivatives, for their ability to induce antigen-specific CD4 and CD8 T cells during Mtb infection. A study reported that aerosol vaccination of RM with AERAS-402, a replication defective adenovirus type 35 that expresses Mtb antigens Ag85A, Ag85B, and TB10.4, induced Ag85A-specific CD4 and CD8 T cells, which produced IFN-γ, TNF-α, and IL-2 but failed to protect against subsequent Mtb challenge. Although the outcome of this study did not support AERAS-402 as an effective vaccine candidate against TB, it suggested that the dose of Mtb used for infection may impact the efficacy of vaccination (Darrah et al. 2014). Another study performed in the RM model reported a protective immunity against pulmonary Mtb infection following aerosol route of vaccination using a mutant Mtb strain defective for *sigH* gene that is involved in bacterial stress response pathway. In this study, elevated accumulation of CD4$^+$ and CD8$^+$ T cells, marked by central memory response in the lungs, was attributed to the improved protection by this vaccine candidate (Kaushal et al. 2015). This study also suggested the presence of iBALT (bronchus-associated lymphoid tissue) to be associated with granuloma formation during Mtb infection. In addition, LAG-3 (lymphocyte activation gene), involved in reducing the Th1-mediated protective immune response, was shown to be highly expressed during pulmonary infection of RM, and silencing of LAG-3 in CD$^+$ T cells enhanced the killing of Mtb and increased the levels of IFN-γ (Phillips et al. 2017).

Latent TB is one of the most concerning states of Mtb infection in humans, since it contributes to reactivation TB, and understanding this stage is important to eradicate bacterial persistence in the host. The formation of Ghon complex, a fibrotic granulomatous nodule with calcified center, is one of the hallmarks of LTBI. This feature is well studied in Mtb-infected CM. In this model, early tubercle/granuloma formation has been shown to be characterized by expression of transcriptional networks controlled by IFN-γ and TNF-α, as well as the intracellular JAK/STAT signaling pathways, indicating potent inflammatory responses. Conversely, later-stage granuloma development was characterized by down-modulation of inflammation and reduced chemokine production. Macaque model has also been used to study LTBI and reactivation during HIV-TB co-infection. The RM model of Mtb-SIV

(Simian Immunodeficiency Virus) co-infection has been shown to mimic the pathological and clinical features of human patients co-infected HIV and Mtb. In this study, SIV infection reactivates TB in RM that was inoculated with either a high dose of BCG or a low dose of a virulent Mtb strain (Shen et al. 2002; Mehra et al. 2011). This reactivation has been shown to be associated with early T cell depletion (Diedrich et al. 2010). These SIV co-infected macaque also expressed lesser amount of pro-inflammatory cytokines, such as IFN-γ and IL-22 as compared to the normal control animals (Guo and Ho 2014). Importantly, anti-retroviral therapy (ART) has been shown to restore Mtb specific T cell immune response in these co-infected RM (Mehra et al. 2011). Consistently, the decreased frequency of CD4$^+$ cells during HIV infection augments the reactivation of TB in AIDS patients and ART reverses the immune response to TB in these patients. In addition, researchers have also investigated a pediatric model of HIV-TB co-infection by infecting newborn macaques with Mtb. This model can help to study TB pathogenesis in children with/without AIDS (Cepeda et al. 2013).

Although the NHP model of TB is immensely useful to understand human disease, this animal species is the most expensive among various animal models. Maintaining NHP colonies and conducting experiments in a relevant biosafety containment facilities pose unique and complicated issues, such as expertise, space, accessibility, and ethical issues that are not common to the other animal models of TB.

Rabbits

Rabbits (*Oryctolagus cuniculus*) are the best animal model, next only to NHP, in recapitulating the pathological features of active and LTBI seen in human cases (Dannenberg 2006). The lung granulomas in Mtb-infected rabbits are of several types and resemble to that found in human disease, including a central necrotic region that undergoes caseation, cavitation, as well as healing and calcification (Dannenberg 2006). Importantly, similar to the necrotic granulomas of pulmonary TB patients, the rabbit lung granulomas are characterized by hypoxia (Haapanen et al. 1959; Via et al. 2008). Moreover, we and others have shown that rabbits display divergent outcome following infection that is dependent on the nature of infecting Mtb strain (Bishai and Chaisson 1999; Manabe et al. 2003; Nedeltchev et al. 2009; Tsenova et al. 2005). Accordingly, aerosol infection of rabbits with a hypervirulent clinical strain of Mtb leads to cavitary disease, while infection by a hyperimmunogenic clinical strain is effectively controlled in the lungs, resulting in LTBI, which can be reactivated by treatment of infected animals with an immune suppressing agent (Subbian et al. 2011a; 2012). These characteristics make rabbit an excellent model for studying the kinetics of Mtb infection toward active TB development or LTBI in humans.

Exposure of rabbits to Mtb-containing aerosol and direct inoculation of Mtb into the trachea have been the standard procedures used to initiate pulmonary infection. We have developed a nose-only aerosol exposure unit and used it to infect rabbits

with the Mtb Beijing strain HN878, a clinical Mtb strain, CDC1551, and a virulent
M. bovis Ravenel strain. The infected animals were studied for the kinetics of
bacterial infection in the lungs over time (Tsenova et al. 2006). Following inoculation of similar numbers of bacteria, a significant difference in bacterial load was
observed at 4 weeks post infection. While the lungs of *M. bovis* Ravenel-infected
rabbits had about 8.5 log_{10} bacteria, the HN878-infected animals had 7 log_{10} bacteria; compared to these, the growth of CDC1551 was significantly reduced (5.5
log_{10}). Similarly, rabbits infected with *M. bovis* Ravenel or HN878 sustained a
higher bacillary load (7–8 log_{10}) until 12 weeks; whereas, the growth of CDC1551
was further reduced by 8 weeks, and no bacilli could be obtained in the infected
rabbit lungs at 16 weeks post infection, thus establishing LTBI (Nedeltchev et al.
2009; Converse et al. 1996). Importantly, treatment of rabbits in the latter group
with corticosteroid led to reactivation of latent infection. Therefore, aerosol infection of rabbits with Mtb-HN878 mimics cavitary, active TB, while Mtb-CDC1551
infection depicts LTBI and reactivation seen in human patients. The histopathology
of lung lesions and their evolution over time were consistent with respective bacillary load in these rabbits; those infected with HN878 had large, necrotic and cavitary lesions with abundant acid-fast bacilli (Subbian et al. 2011a). In contrast, only
few well-developed granulomas were seen in the lungs of CDC1551-infected rabbits that had no necrosis and resorbed by 12 weeks post infection (Subbian et al.
2012). The histopathological finds were also corroborated and extended by immune
cell analysis of the lungs and spleen and also by genome-wide transcriptome profiling of rabbit lungs with active TB or LTBI (Subbian et al. 2011a).

Several studies on the pharmacokinetic (PK) and pharmacodynamic (PD) characteristics of standard antibiotics and novel combination of drugs for TB treatment
have been conducted in the rabbit model of Mtb infection, due primarily to the
nature of lung granulomas that closely resembles the human counterparts; these
lesions cannot be produced in a standard mouse model (Via et al. 2008). Such studies contributed valuable insights on the disparity in drug distribution between blood
(systemic) and local (lung) compartments and revealed the drug efficacy at the site
of infection. A study on the distribution of standard anti-TB drugs, including isoniazid, rifampicin, pyrazinamide, and moxifloxacin, in a rabbit model showed lower
exposures of all drugs, except for moxifloxacin, in the granulomas than in the
plasma (Kjellsson et al. 2012). Similarly, albino rabbits were used to evaluate the
liver toxicity of an anti-TB regimen containing ciprofloxacin, isoniazid, and rifampicin; this study found that ciprofloxacin neither affected the PK/PD of the other
two antibiotics nor increased hepatotoxicity in treated animals (Padilha et al. 2012).
Furthermore, we have shown that adjunctive immune-modulating therapy with an
analog of thalidomide (CC-3052 and CC-11050) in combination with isoniazid
improved bacillary clearance and lung pathology in rabbits with active pulmonary
TB when compared to isoniazid alone (Subbian et al. 2011b, c).

Rabbits are ideal model for studies involving TB pathogenesis and for investigating intervention therapies (Fig. 2). They are smaller and cost effective than NHP, yet
can yield the heterogeneous granulomatous response similar to humans. However,
compared to mouse and NHP models, there is paucity in commercially available,
validated antibodies to study detailed immune response in rabbits. This situation is

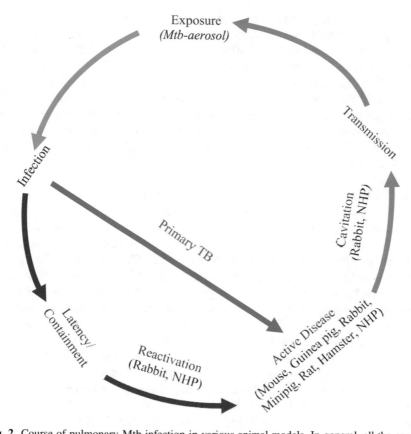

Fig. 2 Course of pulmonary Mtb infection in various animal models. In general, all the experimental animal models of Mtb infection develop active, progressive disease in the lungs following aerosol challenge that are similar to the primary active TB seen in humans. Few animal models develop latency and reactivation that result in active disease. Similarly, few animal models produce cavitary lesions that facilitate disease and pathogen transmission within and out of the infected host. Different stages of Mtb infection/disease progression are denoted in red color letters, and various animal models are shown in black letters. Infection that results in primary TB is denoted by green lines. Infection that results in latency and reactivation is denoted by purple lines. Active disease that progresses to cavitation and transmission is denoted by gray lines

compensated by recently developed technologies such as RNAseq and mRNA-FISH, which enable genome-wide immune correlates associated with severity of disease in Mtb-infected rabbits.

Guinea Pigs

Guinea pigs (*Cavia porcellus*) are the classical model for TB as its use dates to early 1900s. In fact, Robert Koch's postulates were based on the experiments conducted in Mtb-infected guinea pigs; TB being an airborne infection was justified by the studies on guinea pig model. Guinea pigs are susceptible to low-dose aerosol Mtb challenge and develop necrotic lung granulomas as seen in human TB patients. In addition, lung granulomas from both primary and secondary Mtb infections were shown to have different morphology in guinea pigs (Flynn 2006; McMurray 2001). Due to their high susceptibility, this model is highly recommended to mimic TB infections in immunosuppressed individuals and in children. Contributions from David McMurray group have been remarkable in the establishment of guinea pigs as effective model of active TB infection. The development of granulomatous structure and cytokine profiling of Mtb-infected guinea pig lungs have been shown to possess the characteristic of human lesions and have yielded important insights on the role of cytokines in granuloma establishment (Flynn 2006).

In Mtb-infected guinea pigs, the infiltrated neutrophils at the infection foci in the lungs are short lived and degenerate to release their hydrolytic enzymes and cell components, which ultimately produce a necrotic center in the granuloma. These components are scavenged by extravasation of immune cells, such as monocytes, macrophages, and T cells, thus forming a classical TB granuloma. The cytokine profile in each lung lobe of Mtb-infected guinea pig was demonstrated to be different at 6 weeks post infection. This suggested varying cell types and structure of granuloma over time that tracks with progression of infection from acute to chronic phase (Ly et al. 2007). Following pulmonary Mtb infection, the characteristic immune cells observed in guinea pig lung granuloma were epithelioid cells, foamy macrophages, and a significantly high CD4[+] T cells and a low number of CD8[+] T cells on the periphery. Guinea pig model TB has provided a functional role for TNF-α from 3 to 6 weeks post infection in activating the alveolar macrophages that contributes to early containment of Mtb infection (Ly et al. 2007). Protein malnutrition in guinea pigs followed by Mtb infection demonstrated impaired immunity and increased bacterial burden. It was shown that lymphocyte proliferation was greatly impaired in these protein malnourished animals upon vaccination with tuberculin (Dai and McMurray 1998). Vaccination studies in guinea pigs using BCG followed by Mtb infection have demonstrated improved host protection with a shift from inflammatory cytokine environment to an anti-inflammatory niche, after 3 weeks post infection, and control of Mtb dissemination from the lungs to other organs (Ly et al. 2007; McMurray et al. 1989). In vitro Mtb infection of recombinant guinea pig fibroblast cell line demonstrated a causal role for increased IFN-γ production and elevated Mtb killing. Differential virulence of pathogenic and nonpathogenic Mtb, in the context of their ability to elicite IFN-γ levels, was demonstrated at cellular and molecular (mRNA) levels in the guinea pig model of TB (Jeevan et al. 2006).

Guinea pigs are good model animals that can provide better insights into TB pathogenesis and vaccine efficacy. However, there is a lack of immunological tools and reagents available to utilize the guinea pig model to its fullest extent. Although guinea pigs are known to develop a strong delayed-type hypersensitivity (DTH) response, they have relatively (compared to mice) poor cell-mediated immunity to Mtb infection. Also, the inherently high susceptibility of guinea pigs to Mtb infection does not favor latent tuberculosis infection and poses challenge in evaluating clinical Mtb isolates of variable virulence.

Hamster

In the early 1900s when guinea pigs were used as model to study Mtb infection in humans, researchers were also exploring other cost-effective and easy to handle animal models. This search gave emergence to the use of hamsters in Mtb infection studies. Three types of hamsters have been explored for TB research – the golden or Syrian hamster (*Cricetus auratus*) (Dennis and Gaboe 1949; Hussel 1951), the European black-bellied hamster (*Cricetus cricelus*) (Dennis and Gaboe 1949), and the gray-striped hamster (*Cricetus griseus*) from North China (Wang and Meng 1951). Syrian hamsters were tested for their susceptibility to infection caused by mycobacterial strains of human or bovine origin after intramuscular or intraperitoneal infection (Jespersen and Bentzon 1964; Prunescu et al. 1979). These hamsters produced granulomas upon pulmonary Mtb infection, and the macrophages in these granulomas were shown to undergo fine structural changes reminiscent of activation (de Arruda and Montenegro 1995; Dumont and Sheldon 1965). The Syrian golden hamsters were also evaluated for their systemic response to BCG inoculation at various doses. While intravenous inoculation of a higher inoculum (10^7 bacteria) caused death in most of animals, a lower inoculum (10^4 bacteria) was tolerated well; these animals survived and showed a positive response to TST, marked with elevated footpad swelling and splenocyte proliferation (Murohashi et al. 1954). Hamsters were found to be highly susceptible to low doses (0.001 mg) of Mtb infection and produced visible lung tubercles within 16–20 days of infection, although these granulomas showed less evidence of necrotic caseation. The higher susceptibility of hamsters, compared to rabbits and mice, and visible bacterial growth in a short duration of time following infection also suggested use of hamsters over in vitro culture models for anti-tubercular drug screening (Gupta and Mathur 1969). Syrian hamsters were infected by intracardial injection of 0.5 mg Mtb H37Rv and treated with different doses of anti-TB drugs (INH, streptomycin) and survival of animals was noted. Results from this study suggest that Syrian hamsters are useful to study early bactericidal effects of potential anti-TB drugs (Gupta and Mathur 1969). Since hamsters are highly susceptible to Mtb infection that quickly progresses to active disease, this model is not ideal to study various stages of immune response to infection. A hamster cheek pouch model of Mtb infection was introduced in the late 1990s. The cheek pouch in hamsters is a skin invagination of oral mucosa and is immunologically challenged area with poor lymphatic drainage and reduced levels of Langerhans cells. In these pouches, Mtb infection produced small granulomatous lesions marked with a delayed immune response (Dumont and Sheldon 1965; de Arruda and Montenegro 1995). In contrast, a study reported in 1945 demonstrated that golden hamsters were resistant to virulent strain of *Mycobacteria* that infect humans (Steenken and Wagley 1945). In this study, hamsters were infected with virulent Mtb strain and tested for skin test (TST) at 24 days post infection, using different concentrations of tuberculin (5% and 10%). However, the infected animals showed no response to TST, suggesting resistance to infection (Eskuchen 1952; Steenken and Wagley 1945). Interestingly, a study suggested that the initial stages of Mtb infection, until 4 weeks post-inoculation, were similar between guinea pigs and hamsters, but they differed in acquiring resistance to the infecting bacilli (Eskuchen 1952; Ratcliffe and Palladino 1953). Inconsistency in the observations among studies using hamster model of Mtb infection, higher susceptibility of the animals to Mtb infection, and lack of proper granuloma formation in comparison with guinea pigs and the paucity in commercially available immunological reagents have led to reduced use of this model for routine TB studies.

Mice

Mice (*Mus musculus*) are popular model animal for Mtb infection studies because of the commercial availability of vast array of immunological tools, inbred facilities generating genetically modified strains, easy handling and manipulation, and cost-effectiveness (Orme 2003). Some of the key concepts in TB pathogenesis, including the role of adaptive immunity and its components in regulating granuloma formation in the lungs, were established using the mouse model of Mtb infection. Different routes of Mtb infection, including aerosol exposure, intra-nasal, intra-tracheal, intra-venous, and intra-peritoneal, have been reported to develop TB in mice. In these models, depending on the nature of bacteria, the genotype of the mouse, and the route of inoculation, the severity of disease and time to establish disease in the lungs vary. A typical aerosol infection that implants about 100 bacilli in the lungs of a common mouse strain, such as C57BL/6 or BALB/C produces clearly visible granulomas with peak bacillary load (~6 log10 CFU) by 4 weeks post infection. Similar levels of lung bacillary load and elevated disease pathology/granuloma structure is maintained for a very long period (~6 months post infection), ultimately leading to death of the infected animal. The role of several host genes involved in resistance/susceptibility to Mtb infection and/or disease has been demonstrated in mice models. For example, lack of superoxide in mice lacking cytosolic p47^{phox} gene may also result in increased bacterial growth and tissue damage (Cooper et al. 2000).

Following Mtb infection, granuloma formation in most of the common mouse strains is characterized by compact cellular aggregation at the site of infection, marked by the presence of CD4 T cells bounded by epithelioid macrophages and CD8 T cells at the periphery. However, the granulomas in these models do not develop necrosis at the center or cavity formation and calcification and therefore limited in its role in understanding the true/real cellular and immunological events underlying granuloma evolution/maintenance and dissemination of bacteria occurring in human conditions. Some of the mouse strains that are commonly used to study Mtb infection are BALB/C, C57BL/6, and B6D2F1 (Basaraba 2008; Koo et al. 2011; North and Jung 2004; Orme 2005). Different mouse strains show striking difference in their degree of susceptibility to Mtb infection. For example, inbred mouse strains such as CBA, DBA/2, C3H, and 129/SvJ are highly susceptible, whereas other strains including, BALB/c and C57BL/6, are relatively more resistant to TB. As compared to DBA/2 and C3H mice, less bacterial load and increased survival rate were reported in BALB/c and C57BL/6 strains of mouse (Gupta and Katoch 2005). Unlike the rabbit and NHP models, none of the mouse model of Mtb infection can produce reliable, natural, and spontaneous LTBI. In contrast, antibiotic therapy after Mtb infection (the Cornell model) has been shown as a way to create LTBI in mice (Shi et al. 2011). Even though this model fails to establish true latent infection, persistence of Mtb has been demonstrated in the mouse model that involves bacterial manipulation of the host adaptive immune response (Srivastava et al. 2016; Wolf et al. 2007). Similarly, numerous PK/PD studies involving standard- and new anti-TB drugs have been performed in various mouse strains. Thus, mouse model TB is a staple screening tool in the field of TB drug discovery (Srivastava and Gumbo 2011; Nuermberger 2017). Recently, new mouse strains have been introduced to model human Mtb infection; one such strain of mouse, C3HeB/FeJ, has been shown to develop necrotic granulomas after pulmonary infection with Mtb (Kramnik 2008). This model has also been used to evaluate the potency of anti-Mtb drugs (Driver et al. 2012). Although this mouse strain is better than most other mouse strains, in mimicking human lung granulomas upon Mtb infection, C3HeB/FeJ mice are hyper-susceptible to Mtb infection and do not produce LTBI. Another recent mouse model of Mtb infection is the humanized mouse, in which pieces of bone marrow, liver, and thymus (BLT) of human origin are implanted into mouse under immune-compromised conditions; a variation in this model had BCG-infected liver transplanted into the animal (Driver et al. 2012; Harper et al. 2012). These recombinant mouse models have been used for Mtb infection successfully and shown to produce necrotic granulomas, presence of human-like T cells in the lung, liver, and spleen (Calderon et al. 2013). Furthermore, this model has also been explored for Mtb-HIV co-infection studies that showed HIV-dependent cytokine profile and elevated TB pathology in co-infected animals (Nusbaum et al. 2016). In this model, disease-determining factors, such as survival of animal and course of infection, duration of transplanted organ survival, and immunological response, have also been studied (Egen et al. 2008, 2011).

Although recent developments in the mouse models of TB, including the application of C3HeB/FeJ and humanized mice, have the potential to shed more light on TB pathogenesis, these mouse strains possess compromised immune system that makes them highly susceptible to Mtb infection. Similarly, several mouse strains are known to develop a strong cell-mediated immunity; however, they have relatively (compared to guinea pigs) poor delayed-type hypersensitivity (DTH) response to Mtb infection. In addition, these novel mouse strains do not establish LTBI, thus limiting the ability of these models to systematic study of the host factors associated with various types of granulomas and respective immune response, as seen in human lungs with active TB. Additionally, the humanized mouse are expensive and require special care and housing conditions, compared to common/standard strains.

Rats

Rats (*Rattus rattus*) have been studied for their susceptibility to Mtb infection, through several comparative studies with other animal models, as well as to understand the host immune response to varying dose of infectious inoculum (Ratcliffe and Palladino 1953; Gray 1961; Duca 1948; Kumashiro 1958; Tobach and Bloch 1955; Metcoff et al. 1949; Kanai and Yanagisawa 1955). Unlike guinea pigs that mounts a strong delayed-type hypersensitivity (DTH) response but poor cell-mediated immunity (CMI) and mice that develop a strong CMI but a poor DTH, the rat models have been claimed to have a balanced DTH-to-CMI response, similar to rabbits, to Mtb infection. In general, rats are thought to be more resistant, compared to guinea pigs and some mouse strains, and produce a rapid immune response toward Mtb infection (Gray 1961). However, in a study that compared 20 white rats and 12 guinea pigs for their response to Mtb infection showed no significant difference in their susceptibility between these two model animals (Engel 1968a). Several strains of rats, including Lewis, nude, Wistar, and American cotton rats (Elwood et al. 2007; Daigeler 1952), have been tested as model animals for TB studies and found to have divergence in their granulomatous response to Mtb infection and disease progression (Sugawara et al. 2004, 2006; Elwood et al. 2007; Gaonkar et al. 2010). While pulmonary infection of cotton rats (*Sigmodon hispidus*) was shown to produce necrotic granulomas, the Wistar and Lewis rat models do not develop necrotic lesions; the disease presentation in these models resembled more of that in standard mouse models of pulmonary TB. Nonetheless, since rats are extensively used in the studies of chronic diseases, an extensive range of immunological reagents are commercially available for this model (Ratcliffe and Palladino 1953; Gray 1961; Duca 1948; Kumashiro 1958; Tobach and Bloch 1955; Metcoff et al. 1949; Kanai and Yanagisawa 1955). Cotton rats are reported to have different mortality rate upon infection with various doses of virulent strain of Mtb (Elwood et al. 2007; Daigeler 1952; Ryzewska 1969; Kato 1970). Rats were also tested for susceptibility to extrapulmonary Mtb infection (Engel 1968a, 1968b). Granuloma formation and cytokine profile during Mtb infection are well studied for various rat strains used in TB research (Elwood et al. 2007). Albino rats were suggested to have a higher susceptibility to pulmonary infections by different types of microbes; tubercle bacilli can super-infect those lesions, which can result in a rapid TB progression (Smith et al. 1930). Therefore, cotton rats have been proposed to be a better model for studying chronic stages of Mtb infections (Elwood et al. 2009). These rats can be made susceptible to Mtb infection by cortisone administration post infection (Michael et al. 1950). However, cotton rats are natural host for filarial nematodes, such as *Litomosoides sigmodontis*, which may influence the outcome of Mtb infection, although the effect of helminth co-infection on Mtb infection progression and corresponding immunological responses are not well characterized in this model (Hubner et al. 2012). Cotton rats have also been tested for the efficacy of BCG vaccination in controlling bacterial survival after Mtb infection; in this study, BCG vaccination was reported to reduce the bacillary burden significantly in the lung and spleen (Smith et al. 1953). Pulmonary infection of cotton rats with Mtb produced a highly cellular granuloma without central necrosis up to 8 weeks of infection. These granulomas are reminiscent of those found in the lungs of Mtb-infected mouse, although with less foamy macrophages, and not that of Mtb-infected guinea pigs (Cardona and Williams 2017; McFarland et al. 2010).

Rats have been widely used as a preclinical model for anti-tuberculosis drug testing/screening to understand the route of consumption, bioavailability, toxicity, drug-distribution across different organs, half-life, excretion from body and for studies to improve the efficacy of existing antibiotics for TB using combinational therapy or conjugate preparation (Hong et al. 2017; Lu et al. 2016; Sharma et al. 2018; Rawal et al. 2017; Marcianes et al. 2017). For example, in a recent study, YH-8, an inhibitor of a serine threonine kinase B (*pknB*) of Mtb that is required for bacterial growth, was evaluated in a rat model for its PK/PD properties (Zhai et al. 2017). Similarly, rats were used for drug–drug interaction studies: a potential anti-TB drug PA-824 and a HIV drug Darunavir were studied for their interactions when used against HIV-TB cases, and it was concluded that when administered in combination, Darunavir reduces the toxicity of PA-824 and extends its half-life (Wang et al. 2018). Other notable anti-TB drugs that are successfully evaluated in the rat model includes, DFC-2; 2,4-diamino-1-phenyl-1,3,5-triazaspiro[5.5]undeca-2,4-dienes; nitrofuranyl methyl piperazine derivative, IIIM-MCD-211; and delamanid (Seo et al. 2018; Yang et al. 2018; Magotra et al. 2018; Shibata et al. 2017).

Recently, rats are also being evaluated as TB detection agents to complement other TB diagnostic systems, such as culture and Xpert MTB/RIF (Mulder et al. 2017b). In this method, African giant pouched rats (*Cricetomys gambianus*) were trained to sniff the scent of heat inactivated sputum samples from suspected pulmonary TB patients (Mulder et al. 2017a). These studies have found that following "sniff training", this strain of rats are capable of identifying TB samples from non-TB, control samples. Rat training was a part of behavioral studies where rats were rewarded for correct identification of TB positive samples (Mulder et al. 2017a). Researchers also studied the reproducibility of TB-positive sample detection by trained rats, compared to standard culture and microscopy methods. Detected positive samples were confirmed using Xpert MTB/RIF and microscopy. In a comparative study, TB positive sample detection by trained rats was reported to be 72–80% more sensitive and 59–74% specific than conventional smear microscopy method. In a study carried out in Tanzania and Mozambique, nearly 12,000 suspected sputum samples from TB clinics were assessed for positivity by sniffing rats (Ellis et al. 2017). Findings from this study support a higher degree of TB detection reproducibility by giant pouched rats that this method was suggested as an independent technique for TB detection (Ellis et al. 2017). However, other studies suggest the use of trained rats in association with microscopy as confirmatory technique (Mulder et al. 2017a; Poling et al. 2015). A recent "rat-sniffing" study conducted with 55,148 presumptive TB sputum samples from pulmonary TB patients in Tanzania showed that TB-positive sputum sample detection by rats was 67.6% more than detection in the clinics using smear microscopy (Mgode et al. 2018). However, this methodology needs more rigorous validation studies, including test samples from different

TB endemic countries; In addition, consistency/reliability and applicability to practical use are some of the challenges method of TB diagnosis.

Marmosets

Although nonhuman primates display highly identical disease progression as humans following Mtb infection, their size, cost, ethical issues, and other unique requirements to conduct studies in NHP limit their use as a high-throughput or routine model for TB studies. Marmosets (*Callithrix jacchus*) are considered an alternate to NHP and have gained popularity due to their small size, ease to handle, and already explored relevance of anatomy and physiology, through other diseases, to human disease conditions. Marmosets were first studied for TB progression and bacterial burden using PET/CT scan methodology at regular intervals post infection with different strains of Mtb complex (Via et al. 2013). In this model, differential virulence was explored; while a low-dose infection with Mtb-CDC1551 was contained with decreased bacterial burden, similar low-dose infection with Mtb-Erdman resulted in severe disease symptoms, such as weight loss and rapid progression of disease pathology (Via et al. 2013). Since marmosets infected with Mtb can produce cavitary lesions in the lungs, this model was also evaluated for anti-TB drug screening study (Via et al. 2015). Thus, marmosets are emerging as an effective model in understanding the immune response to different types of infecting Mtb strains. Furthermore, marmoset model of Mtb infection was studied for reducing the duration of current anti-TB drug regimen (Via et al. 2015). In a comparative study, the efficacy of using a combination of four drugs, isoniazid, pyrazinamide, ethambutol, and rifampicin, was evaluated against a two-drug regimen of isoniazid and streptomycin. This study showed similar level of reduction in lung bacterial load by both of the tested anti-TB regimens after 6 weeks of treatment (Via et al. 2015).

Although marmosets are deemed as small animal model and appear to be a better alternate to NHP, they are more susceptible to Mtb infection, similar to guinea pigs and some mouse strains that produce necrotic granulomas. In addition, requirement of specialized equipment for manipulation and housing, lack of availability of validated immunological reagents, and relatively high cost, compared to mice, guinea pigs, and rabbits, limit the application of this model for routine and elaborate TB studies.

Minipigs

Minipig (*Sus scrofa domesticus*) model of Mtb infection has been established very recently, and only a few groups have conducted experiments in this model (Gil et al. 2010; Ramos et al. 2017). Low-dose inoculation of Mtb through transthoracic route was shown to produce latent infection in minipigs that resembles human

LTBI condition, including the presence of a fibrotic encapsulation of healing granulomas and a positive correlation between Th1 response and containment of disease in the lungs (Gil et al. 2010). Infected minipigs also responded positively to anti-TB therapy, showing a reduction in bacterial CFU count and dissemination ratio and calcification of lesions where non-replicating Mtb was present. In another study, minipigs were explored as a model to represent TB in childhood, adolescent, and adult stages. In this model, aerosol infection of minipigs with Mtb at different ages (corresponding to respective growth stages in humans) was followed for up to 36 weeks post infection. Results of this study claim that minipigs infected with Mtb produce lung pathology and disease similar to human patients at different age/level of development. In addition, this study also claims that minipigs can be a good model to study natural transmission of TB. Since minipigs are commonly used to study diseases, such as Alzheimer and diabetes, many immunological reagents are commercially available for this model. In addition, the key features of minipig immune system have been successfully characterized and its genome sequenced. However, this model is relatively new and needs to be developed further to understand the host–pathogen interactions to Mtb infection in a elaborate and systematic fashion.

Zebrafish

Zebrafish (*Danio rerio*) has a transparent body system when they are young that allows visualizing and imaging the internal organs efficiently, in live animals. Therefore, zebrafish as a model organism has the advantage of interrogating prominent host–pathogen interactions during Mtb infection in real time using optical imaging systems. Since Mtb of human origin do not infect zebrafish, a surrogate of virulent *Mycobacteria*, *M. marinum*, also a natural pathogen of zebrafish, has been used for infection in this model. Genetically, *M. marinum* closely resembles Mtb, although the former has shorter generation time (4 h vs ~24 h for Mtb), requires lower temperature for optimal growth (~18–20 °C vs 37 °C for Mtb), and does not require BSL3 biosafety measures (work can be carried out at BSL2 facility). Despite these differences, *M. marinum* infection causes TB-like disease with granuloma formation, mainly in cold-blooded animals. Zebrafish can be challenged with *M. marinum* via various inoculation routes such as intraperitoneal or intramuscular injection. In addition, injection of bacteria into the yolk of embryo is an alternative method applied in high-throughput studies (Meijer and Spaink 2011; Cronan and Tobin 2014). Zebrafish infection models have been explored to understand the early stages of granuloma formation and have been a useful tool in explaining the dissemination of *Mycobacteria* to form secondary granulomas (Rubin 2009; Oksanen et al. 2013). The optical transparency of zebrafish larva model has provided visualization of *M. marinum* infection from invasion of macrophages by bacteria to macrophage recruitment at the site of infection to form granuloma-like structures (Davis et al. 2002).

In the zebrafish model of TB, two different infection systems have been developed: an adult fish model and an embryonic larvae model. Adult zebrafish model demonstrates innate and adaptive immune markers that are similar to human and mouse Mtb infection model, whereas larval stage lacks adaptive immune response and represents only the innate phase of immunity. The zebrafish model of mycobacterial infection can lead to either latent or active disease, depending on the infectious dose and strain of bacteria used for the infection. Following mycobacterial infection of adult zebrafish, the granulomas develop in fatty tissues of several organs including liver, adipose tissue, spleen, and gonads (Oksanen et al. 2013; Parikka et al. 2012; Stoop et al. 2013). Adult zebrafish model mimics the pathological features and immune response of other animal models of TB, where the adaptive immunity develops after 3–4 weeks of infection. One of the key advantages of zebrafish model is that it develops necrotic granulomas with cellular cuff that separates them from the surrounding tissues after 16–20 weeks post infection (Parikka et al. 2012; Ramakrishnan et al. 2012; Berg and Ramakrishnan 2012). Similar to humans, a fully developed adaptive immunity is required to control the infection in zebrafish. A low-dose *M. marinum* inoculation develops latent infection in zebrafish; radiation-mediated immune suppression treatment induces reactivation of disease by depleting immune cells in these animals (Parikka et al. 2012). This suggests that zebrafish model can be used to study determinants of mycobacterial dormancy, latency, and clinical manifestation of disease reactivation. Zebrafish model of infection has also shown that Th2 type immune cells help to maintain the balance in immune response during infection and contributes to restrict mycobacterial growth (Hammarén et al. 2014).

The embryonic model has been shown to be useful to study early mycobacterial pathogenesis and innate immune response (4–6 days) (Ramakrishnan 2013; Yang et al. 2012). In this model, real-time imaging studies revealed that macrophages phagocytose the bacteria and cross both endothelial and epithelial barriers to form granuloma-like infectious clusters (Tobin and Ramakrishnan 2008; Lesley and Ramakrishnan 2008). This difference in immune development from larval to adult has also been exploited to understand the role of macrophages and TNF-α in the formation of granuloma like-cellular aggregates and maintaining its integrity during chronic mycobacterial infection (Clay et al. 2008; Oksanen et al. 2013). However, formation of granuloma-like aggregates was also noticed in infected zebrafish mutant embryos with underdeveloped thymus, thus lacking T lymphocytes (Davis et al. 2002). By creating morphants lacking macrophages, the role of macrophages in engulfing *Mycobacteria* and forming granuloma-like structures was further established, since these morphants had increased bacterial burden in tissues (Clay et al. 2007). This study highlights the role of innate immune response, particularly of macrophages in early granuloma formation. In addition, zebrafish model of infection was used to study the dynamics of granuloma maturation and evolution. Studies revealed that in this model, the infected macrophages detach from granulomas and move to new location within and out of the infected tissue to form secondary granulomas (Ramakrishnan 2013).

Zebrafish infection models have been extensively explored to determine the role of several mycobacterial virulence determinants that affect pathogenesis, including phagocyte recruitment to the site of infection. For example, successful *M. marinum* infection of zebrafish is independent of MyD88, a downstream adaptor of TLR signaling, whereas deletion of MyD88 leads to a decrease in macrophage recruitment following infection with *M. smegmatis, Staphylococcus aureus,* and *Pseudomonas aeruginosa* (Cambier et al. 2014). Similarly, lipids of *Mycobacteria* such as PDIM and PGL were demonstrated to influence the host immune mechanisms in the zebrafish model; PDIM was shown to mask pathogen-associated molecular patterns (PAMPs), thus inhibiting TLR signaling that subsequently impairs recruitment of macrophage and their production of reactive nitrogen species. On the other hand, PGL was shown to facilitate CCR2-mediated macrophage recruitment (Cambier et al. 2014). Similarly, the role of a mycobacterial peptidoglycan hydrolase, MarP, was demonstrated in zebrafish model, in which it was shown that MarP provides lysosomal acid tolerance to the bacteria after phagocytosis, thus promoting intracellular mycobacterial growth (Levitte et al. 2016). The zebrafish model was used to demonstrate the role of one of the virulent islands of *Mycobacteria*, RD-1, and a mycobacterial secretion system, ESX-1, in promoting granuloma formation by recruiting macrophages to the site of infection through induction of host cell matrix metalloprotease-9 (Pagan et al. 2015; Volkman et al. 2004; Volkman et al. 2010; Gao et al. 2004). Recently, a study reported the significance of mycobacterial SecA2 secretion system in granuloma formation using the zebrafish model (Watkins et al. 2012). Thousands of transposon mutants of pathogenic *Mycobacteria* were screened in the zebrafish model to identify virulent genes important for establishment of infection (Stoop et al. 2011, 2013; van der Woude et al. 2014). Zebrafish embryo model has also been used to study the role of host genetics in the susceptibility to mycobacterial infection. As noticed in human population, zebrafish with mutations in the *lta4h* locus that codes for a leukotriene A4 hydrolase were more susceptible to *M. marinum* infection. This mutation has been shown to cause loss of immune balance and subsequent exacerbated inflammation that result in tissue damage (Tobin et al. 2010, 2012). Similarly, *M. marinum* infection of zebrafish embryo that has defective *ptpn6* (protein tyrosine phosphatase non-receptor type 6) gene resulted in the downregulation of inflammation caused by infection (Kanwal et al. 2013).

Although the zebrafish model has provided details on the mechanism of mycobacterial entry into macrophages and cellular organization during infection, it differs strikingly in its response to mycobacterial infection and the type of granuloma formation, compared to other mammalian models of TB. Also, a major disadvantage accompanied with this model is the significant dissimilarity in physiology and anatomy between mammalian systems, such as a lack of lung structure in the zebrafish model. This makes it harder to understand the relevance, context, and extension of the findings made in zebrafish model to apply directly to the pathogenesis of human TB.

Summary and Conclusion

Animal models of Mtb infection/TB have played a crucial role in providing insight into the in vivo environment to researchers for better understanding of the host-pathogen interactions during the course of infection. Right from the mode of infection to pathogenesis of disease and ultimately to its transmission, animal models have established a significant amount of knowledge in TB research that we have today (Fig. 1). They have been beneficial in exploring immunological tools and diagnostic techniques, and they have been widely used for testing new vaccine candidates, anti-mycobacterial drugs, and new regimen for treatment. Animal models have contributed significantly to our understanding of various immune cell types, their function and interaction as well as relevence to active or latent TB in humans. However, eradication of TB still stands as the far-fetched target for researchers. Although animal models have shown us stages of infection and immunological response, they have also introduced us with the fact that host-dependent immune response towards an infection can differ strikingly within and between various species. While guinea pig and rabbit models of Mtb infection have demonstrated relatively human-like disease progression and granuloma formation, the guinea pig model fails to correlate with the latent tuberculosis infection and associated immunological responses. Similarly, the NHPs have more genetic resemblance with human and display human-like granuloma formation; however, the expense and need for highly skilled professional and infrastructure have limited their use to only few institutions. Minipigs and marmosets have limited immunological reagents available and are expensive and difficult to handle. On the other hand, mouse models, which have been extensively used in creating immunological tools for TB research and easy to genetically manipulate and handle, failed to form necrotic caseating and cavitary granulomas as well as LTBI, two key aspects of pulmonary Mtb infection in humans. Further complicating the comparative analysis of animals to humans, drug-resistant Mtb strains have urged the need for development of new treatment regimen targetting the host-directed factors. However, variations in the host response seen in different animal models upon infection with the same pathogen, have developed divergence in beliefs on the fate of granuloma formation and the course of Mtb infection. Therefore, no single animal model stands out as a perfect model to study all aspects of the human disease, and need for a proper study design still remains as a key tool for developing better diagnosis, vaccine candidates and anti-TB drugs that are capable of eradicating the disease.

References

Basaraba, R. J. (2008). Experimental tuberculosis: The role of comparative pathology in the discovery of improved tuberculosis treatment strategies. *Tuberculosis (Edinburgh, Scotland), 88*(Suppl 1), S35–S47.

Berg, R. D., & Ramakrishnan, L. (2012). Insights into tuberculosis from the zebrafish model. *Trends in Molecular Medicine, 18*(12), 689 690.

Bishai, W. R., & Chaisson, R. E. (1999). Opportunistic infections: Down but not out. *The Hopkins HIV Report, 11*(2), 2, 7, 12.

Calderon, V. E., Valbuena, G., Goez, Y., Judy, B. M., Huante, M. B., Sutjita, P., et al. (2013). A humanized mouse model of tuberculosis. *PLoS One, 8*(5), e63331.

Cambier, C. J., Takaki, K. K., Larson, R. P., Hernandez, R. E., Tobin, D. M., Urdahl, K. B., et al. (2014). *Mycobacteria* manipulate macrophage recruitment through coordinated use of membrane lipids. *Nature, 505*(7482), 218–222.

Capuano, S. V., 3rd, Croix, D. A., Pawar, S., Zinovik, A., Myers, A., Lin, P. L., et al. (2003). Experimental *Mycobacterium tuberculosis* infection of cynomolgus macaques closely resembles the various manifestations of human *M. tuberculosis* infection. *Infection and Immunity, 71*(10), 5831–5844.

Cardona, P. J., & Williams, A. (2017). Experimental animal modelling for TB vaccine development. *International Journal of Infectious Diseases, 56*, 268–273.

Carlsson, F., Kim, J., Dumitru, C., Barck, K. H., Carano, R. A., Sun, M., et al. (2010). Host-detrimental role of Esx-1-mediated inflammasome activation in mycobacterial infection. *PLoS Pathogens, 6*(5), e1000895.

Cepeda, M., Salas, M., Folwarczny, J., Leandro, A. C., Hodara, V. L., de la Garza, M. A., et al. (2013). Establishment of a neonatal rhesus macaque model to study *Mycobacterium tuberculosis* infection. *Tuberculosis (Edinburgh, Scotland)*, (93 Suppl), S51–S59.

Clay, H., Davis, J. M., Beery, D., Huttenlocher, A., Lyons, S. E., & Ramakrishnan, L. (2007). Dichotomous role of the macrophage in early *Mycobacterium marinum* infection of the zebrafish. *Cell Host & Microbe, 2*(1), 29–39.

Clay, H., Volkman, H. E., & Ramakrishnan, L. (2008). Tumor necrosis factor signaling mediates resistance to mycobacteria by inhibiting bacterial growth and macrophage death. *Immunity, 29*(2), 283–294.

Converse, P. J., Dannenberg, A. M., Jr., Estep, J. E., Sugisaki, K., Abe, Y., Schofield, B. H., et al. (1996). Cavitary tuberculosis produced in rabbits by aerosolized virulent tubercle bacilli. *Infection and Immunity, 64*(11), 4776–4787.

Cooper, A. M., Segal, B. H., Frank, A. A., Holland, S. M., & Orme, I. M. (2000). Transient loss of resistance to pulmonary tuberculosis in p47(phox-/-) mice. *Infection and Immunity, 68*(3), 1231–1234.

Cronan, M. R., & Tobin, D. M. (2014). Fit for consumption: Zebrafish as a model for tuberculosis. *Disease Models & Mechanisms, 7*(7), 777–784.

Dai, G., & McMurray, D. N. (1998). Altered cytokine production and impaired antimycobacterial immunity in protein-malnourished guinea pigs. *Infection and Immunity, 66*(8), 3562–3568.

Daigeler, A. (1952). The cotton rat (*Sigmodon hispidus* hispidus) as an experimental animal in the diagnosis of tuberculosis. *Zeitschrift für Hygiene und Infektionskrankheiten, 135*(6), 588–591.

Dannenberg, A. M., Jr. (2006). *Pathogenesis of human pulmonary tuberculosis: Insights from the rabbit model*. Washington, DC: ASM Press. xiv + 453 pp.

Darrah, P. A., Bolton, D. L., Lackner, A. A., Kaushal, D., Aye, P. P., Mehra, S., et al. (2014). Aerosol vaccination with AERAS-402 elicits robust cellular immune responses in the lungs of rhesus macaques but fails to protect against high-dose *Mycobacterium tuberculosis* challenge. *Journal of Immunology (Baltimore, MD: 1950), 193*(4), 1799–1811.

Davis, J. M., Clay, H., Lewis, J. L., Ghori, N., Herbomel, P., & Ramakrishnan, L. (2002). Real-time visualization of *Mycobacterium*-macrophage interactions leading to initiation of granuloma formation in zebrafish embryos. *Immunity, 17*(6), 693–702.

de Arruda, M. S., & Montenegro, M. R. (1995). The hamster cheek pouch: An immunologically privileged site suitable to the study of granulomatous infections. *Revista do Instituto de Medicina Tropical de São Paulo, 37*(4), 303–309.

Dennis, E. W., & Gaboe, F. C. (1949). Experimental tuberculosis of the Syrian hamster, Cricetus auratus. *Annals of the New York Academy of Sciences, 52*(5), 646–661, incl 2 pl.

Diedrich, C. R., Mattila, J. T., Klein, E., Janssen, C., Phuah, J., Sturgeon, T. J., et al. (2010). Reactivation of latent tuberculosis in cynomolgus macaques infected with SIV is associated with early peripheral T cell depletion and not virus load. *PLoS One, 5*(3), e9611.

Driver, E. R., Ryan, G. J., Hoff, D. R., Irwin, S. M., Basaraba, R. J., Kramnik, I., et al. (2012). Evaluation of a mouse model of necrotic granuloma formation using C3HeB/FeJ mice for testing of drugs against *Mycobacterium tuberculosis*. *Antimicrobial Agents and Chemotherapy, 56*(6), 3181–3195.

Duca, C. J. (1948). Age specific susceptibility to tuberculosis; experiments on guinea pigs and rats. *American Review of Tuberculosis, 57*(4), 389–399.

Dumont, A., & Sheldon, H. (1965). Changes in the fine structure of macrophages in experimentally produced tuberculous granulomas in hamsters. *Laboratory Investigation, 14*(11), 2034–2055.

Egen, J. G., Rothfuchs, A. G., Feng, C. G., Winter, N., Sher, A., & Germain, R. N. (2008). Macrophage and T cell dynamics during the development and disintegration of mycobacterial granulomas. *Immunity, 28*(2), 271–284.

Egen, J. G., Rothfuchs, A. G., Feng, C. G., Horwitz, M. A., Sher, A., & Germain, R. N. (2011). Intravital imaging reveals limited antigen presentation and T cell effector function in mycobacterial granulomas. *Immunity, 34*(5), 807–819.

Ellis, H., Mulder, C., Valverde, E., Poling, A., & Edwards, T. (2017). Reproducibility of African giant pouched rats detecting Mycobacterium tuberculosis. *BMC Infectious Diseases, 17*(1), 298.

Elwood, R. L., Wilson, S., Blanco, J. C., Yim, K., Pletneva, L., Nikonenko, B., et al. (2007). The American cotton rat: A novel model for pulmonary tuberculosis. *Tuberculosis (Edinburgh, Scotland), 87*(2), 145–154.

Elwood, R. L., Rajnik, M., Wilson, S., Yim, K., Blanco, J. C., Nikonenko, B., et al. (2009). Characterization of late tuberculosis infection in *Sigmodon hispidus*. *Tuberculosis (Edinburgh, Scotland), 89*(2), 183–188.

Engel, D. (1968a). The influence of the biochemical milieu on the development of tubercles in the testis and epididymis. *Beiträge zur Klinik und Erforschung der Tuberkulose und der Lungenkrankheiten, 137*(4), 353–370.

Engel, D. (1968b). The practical significance of the chemical milieu for the course of tuberculosis of the male genital organs. *Urologia Internationalis, 23*(4), 356–363.

Eskuchen. (1952). Diagnosis of tuberculosis with guinea pigs and gold hamster. *Der Tuberkulosearzt, 6*(6), 356–358.

Flynn, J. L. (2006). Lessons from experimental *Mycobacterium tuberculosis* infections. *Microbes and Infection, 8*(4), 1179–1188.

Flynn, R., Grundmann, A., Renz, P., Hanseler, W., James, W. S., Cowley, S. A., et al. (2015). CRISPR-mediated genotypic and phenotypic correction of a chronic granulomatous disease mutation in human iPS cells. *Experimental Hematology, 43*(10), 838–48.e3.

Gao, L. Y., Guo, S., McLaughlin, B., Morisaki, H., Engel, J. N., & Brown, E. J. (2004). A mycobacterial virulence gene cluster extending RD1 is required for cytolysis, bacterial spreading and ESAT-6 secretion. *Molecular Microbiology, 53*(6), 1677–1693.

Gaonkar, S., Bharath, S., Kumar, N., Balasubramanian, V., & Shandil, R. K. (2010). Aerosol infection model of tuberculosis in wistar rats. *International Journal of Microbiology, 2010*, 426035.

Gil, O., Diaz, I., Vilaplana, C., Tapia, G., Diaz, J., Fort, M., et al. (2010). Granuloma encapsulation is a key factor for containing tuberculosis infection in minipigs. *PLoS One, 5*(4), e10030.

Gray, D. F. (1961). The relative natural resistance of rats and mice to experimental pulmonary tuberculosis. *Journal of Hygiene (London), 59*, 471–477.

Green, J. A., Rand, L., Moores, R., Dholakia, S., Pezas, T., Elkington, P. T., et al. (2013). In an in vitro model of human tuberculosis, monocyte-microglial networks regulate matrix metalloproteinase-1 and -3 gene expression and secretion via a p38 mitogen activated protein kinase-dependent pathway. *Journal of Neuroinflammation, 10*, 107.

Guo, M., & Ho, W. Z. (2014). Animal models to study *Mycobacterium tuberculosis* and HIV co-infection. *Dong wu xue yan jiu = Zoological Research, 35*(3), 163–169.

Gupta, U. D., & Katoch, V. M. (2005). Animal models of tuberculosis. *Tuberculosis (Edinburgh, Scotland), 85*(5–6), 277–293.

Gupta, S. K., & Mathur, I. S. (1969). A cheap and quick method of screening potential antimycobacterial agents in the Syrian or golden hamster (Cricetus auratus). *Experientia, 25*(7), 782–783.

Haapanen, J. H., Kass, I., Gensini, G., & Middlebrook, G. (1959). Studies on the gaseous content of tuberculous cavities. *The American review of respiratory disease, 80*(1, Part 1), 1–5.

Hammarén, M. M., Oksanen, K. E., Nisula, H. M., Luukinen, B. V., Pesu, M., Rämet, M., et al. (2014). Adequate Th2-type response associates with restricted bacterial growth in latent mycobacterial infection of zebrafish. *PLoS Pathogens, 10*(6), e1004190.

Harper, J., Skerry, C., Davis, S. L., Tasneen, R., Weir, M., Kramnik, I., et al. (2012). Mouse model of necrotic tuberculosis granulomas develops hypoxic lesions. *The Journal of Infectious Diseases, 205*(4), 595–602.

Hong, W. D., Gibbons, P. D., Leung, S. C., Amewu, R., Stocks, P. A., Stachulski, A., et al. (2017). Rational design, synthesis, and biological evaluation of heterocyclic quinolones targeting the respiratory chain of *Mycobacterium tuberculosis*. *Journal of Medicinal Chemistry, 60*(9), 3703–3726.

Hubner, M. P., Killoran, K. E., Rajnik, M., Wilson, S., Yim, K. C., Torrero, M. N., et al. (2012). Chronic helminth infection does not exacerbate *Mycobacterium tuberculosis* infection. *PLoS Neglected Tropical Diseases, 6*(12), e1970.

Hussel, L. (1951). [Suitability of the golden hamster as laboratory animal in tuberculosis diagnosis]. Zentralblatt fur Bakteriologie, Parasitenkunde, Infektionskrankheiten und Hygiene 1 Abt Medizinisch-hygienische Bakteriologie, Virusforschung und Parasitologie. *Originale, 156*(6), 445–450.

Janicki, B. W., Good, R. C., Minden, P., Affronti, L. F., & Hymes, W. F. (1973). Immune responses in rhesus monkeys after bacillus Calmette-Guerin vaccination and aerosol challenge with *Mycobacterium tuberculosis*. *The American Review of Respiratory Disease, 107*(3), 359–366.

Jeevan, A., McFarland, C. T., Yoshimura, T., Skwor, T., Cho, H., Lasco, T., et al. (2006). Production and characterization of guinea pig recombinant gamma interferon and its effect on macrophage activation. *Infection and Immunity, 74*(1), 213–224.

Jespersen, A., & Bentzon, M. W. (1964). The virulence of various strains of BCG determined on the golden hamster. *Acta Tuberculosea et Pneumologica Scandinavica, 44*, 222–249.

Kanai, K., & Yanagisawa, K. (1955). Studies on the reinfection in experimental tuberculosis of rats. *Japanese Journal of Medical Science & Biology, 8*(2), 129–134.

Kanwal, Z., Zakrzewska, A., den Hertog, J., Spaink, H. P., Schaaf, M. J., & Meijer, A. H. (2013). Deficiency in hematopoietic phosphatase ptpn6/Shp1 hyperactivates the innate immune system and impairs control of bacterial infections in zebrafish embryos. *Journal of Immunology (Baltimore, MD: 1950), 190*(4), 1631–1645.

Kato, M. (1970). Site II-specific inhibition of mitochondria oxidative phosphorylation by trehalose-6,6′-dimycolate (cord factor) of *Mycobacterium tuberculosis*. *Archives of Biochemistry and Biophysics, 140*(2), 379–390.

Kaushal, D., Foreman, T. W., Gautam, U. S., Alvarez, X., Adekambi, T., Rangel-Moreno, J., et al. (2015). Mucosal vaccination with attenuated *Mycobacterium tuberculosis* induces strong central memory responses and protects against tuberculosis. *Nature Communications, 6*, 8533.

Kita, Y., Hashimoto, S., Nakajima, T., Nakatani, H., Nishimatsu, S., Nishida, Y., et al. (2013). Novel therapeutic vaccines [(HSP65 + IL-12)DNA-, granulysin- and Ksp37-vaccine] against tuberculosis and synergistic effects in the combination with chemotherapy. *Human Vaccines & Immunotherapeutics, 9*(3), 526–533.

Kjellsson, M. C., Via, L. E., Goh, A., Weiner, D., Low, K. M., Kern, S., et al. (2012). Pharmacokinetic evaluation of the penetration of antituberculosis agents in rabbit pulmonary lesions. *Antimicrobial Agents and Chemotherapy, 56*(1), 446–457.

Koo, M.-S., Manca, C., Yang, G., O'Brien, P., Sung, N., Tsenova, L., et al. (2011). Phosphodiesterase 4 inhibition reduces innate immunity and improves isoniazid clearance of *Mycobacterium tuberculosis* in the lungs of infected mice. *PLoS One, 6*(2), e17091.

Kramnik, I. (2008). Genetic dissection of host resistance to *Mycobacterium tuberculosis*: The sst1 locus and the Ipr1 gene. *Current Topics in Microbiology and Immunology, 321*, 123–148.

Kumashiro, A. (1958). Study on the susceptibility of rats to various strains of mycobacteria. III. The humoral defensive power of rats against mycobacteria. *Acta Tuberculosea Japonica, 8*(1–2), 22–31.

Langermans, J. A., Andersen, P., van Soolingen, D., Vervenne, R. A., Frost, P. A., van der Laan, T., et al. (2001). Divergent effect of bacillus Calmette-Guerin (BCG) vaccination on *Mycobacterium tuberculosis* infection in highly related macaque species: Implications for primate models in tuberculosis vaccine research. *Proceedings of the National Academy of Sciences of the United States of America, 98*(20), 11497–11502.

Larsen, M. H., Biermann, K., Chen, B., Hsu, T., Sambandamurthy, V. K., Lackner, A. A., et al. (2009). Efficacy and safety of live attenuated persistent and rapidly cleared *Mycobacterium tuberculosis* vaccine candidates in non-human primates. *Vaccine, 27*(34), 4709–4717.

Lesley, R., & Ramakrishnan, L. (2008). Insights into early mycobacterial pathogenesis from the zebrafish. *Current Opinion in Microbiology, 11*(3), 277–283.

Levitte, S., Adams, K. N., Berg, R. D., Cosma, C. L., Urdahl, K. B., & Ramakrishnan, L. (2016). Mycobacterial acid tolerance enables phagolysosomal survival and establishment of tuberculous infection in vivo. *Cell Host & Microbe, 20*(2), 250–258.

Lin, P. L., Pawar, S., Myers, A., Pegu, A., Fuhrman, C., Reinhart, T. A., et al. (2006). Early events in *Mycobacterium tuberculosis* infection in cynomolgus macaques. *Infection and Immunity, 74*(7), 3790–3803.

Lin, P. L., Rodgers, M., Smith, L., Bigbee, M., Myers, A., Bigbee, C., et al. (2009). Quantitative comparison of active and latent tuberculosis in the cynomolgus macaque model. *Infection and Immunity, 77*(10), 4631–4642.

Lin, P. L., Myers, A., Smith, L., Bigbee, C., Bigbee, M., Fuhrman, C., et al. (2010). Tumor necrosis factor neutralization results in disseminated disease in acute and latent *Mycobacterium tuberculosis* infection with normal granuloma structure in a cynomolgus macaque model. *Arthritis and Rheumatism, 62*(2), 340–350.

Lin, P. L., Dietrich, J., Tan, E., Abalos, R. M., Burgos, J., Bigbee, C., et al. (2012). The multistage vaccine H56 boosts the effects of BCG to protect cynomolgus macaques against active tuberculosis and reactivation of latent *Mycobacterium tuberculosis* infection. *The Journal of Clinical Investigation, 122*(1), 303–314.

Lin, P. L., Coleman, T., Carney, J. P., Lopresti, B. J., Tomko, J., Fillmore, D., et al. (2013). Radiologic responses in cynomolgus macaques for assessing tuberculosis chemotherapy regimens. *Antimicrobial Agents and Chemotherapy, 57*(9), 4237–4244.

Lu, X., Tang, J., Liu, Z., Li, M., Zhang, T., Zhang, X., et al. (2016). Discovery of new chemical entities as potential leads against *Mycobacterium tuberculosis*. *Bioorganic & Medicinal Chemistry Letters, 26*(24), 5916–5919.

Luciw, P. A., Oslund, K. L., Yang, X. W., Adamson, L., Ravindran, R., Canfield, D. R., et al. (2011). Stereological analysis of bacterial load and lung lesions in nonhuman primates (rhesus macaques) experimentally infected with *Mycobacterium tuberculosis*. *American Journal of Physiology. Lung Cellular and Molecular Physiology, 301*(5), L731–L738.

Ly, L. H., Russell, M. I., & McMurray, D. N. (2007). Microdissection of the cytokine milieu of pulmonary granulomas from tuberculous guinea pigs. *Cellular Microbiology, 9*(5), 1127–1136.

Magalhaes, I., Sizemore, D. R., Ahmed, R. K., Mueller, S., Wehlin, L., Scanga, C., et al. (2008). rBCG induces strong antigen-specific T cell responses in rhesus macaques in a prime-boost setting with an adenovirus 35 tuberculosis vaccine vector. *PLoS One, 3*(11), e3790.

Magotra, A., Sharma, A., Singh, S., Ojha, P. K., Kumar, S., Bokolia, N., et al. (2018). Physicochemical, pharmacokinetic, efficacy and toxicity profiling of a potential nitrofuranyl methyl piperazine derivative IIIM-MCD-211 for oral tuberculosis therapy via in-silico-in-vitro-in-vivo approach. *Pulmonary Pharmacology & Therapeutics, 48*, 151–160.

Maiello, P., DiFazio, R. M., Cadena, A. M., Rodgers, M. A., Lin, P. L., Scanga, C. A., et al. (2018). Rhesus macaques are more susceptible to progressive tuberculosis than cynomolgus macaques: A quantitative comparison. *Infection and Immunity, 86*(2), pii: e00505-17.

Manabe, Y. C., Dannenberg, A. M., Jr., Tyagi, S. K., Hatem, C. L., Yoder, M., Woolwine, S. C., et al. (2003). Different strains of *Mycobacterium tuberculosis* cause various spectrums of disease in the rabbit model of tuberculosis. *Infection and Immunity, 71*(10), 6004–6011.

Marcianes, P., Negro, S., Garcia-Garcia, L., Montejo, C., Barcia, E., & Fernandez-Carballido, A. (2017). Surface-modified gatifloxacin nanoparticles with potential for treating central nervous system tuberculosis. *International Journal of Nanomedicine, 12*, 1959–1968.

Mattila, J. T., Ojo, O. O., Kepka-Lenhart, D., Marino, S., Kim, J. H., Eum, S. Y., et al. (2013). Microenvironments in tuberculous granulomas are delineated by distinct populations of macrophage subsets and expression of nitric oxide synthase and arginase isoforms. *Journal of Immunology (Baltimore, MD: 1950), 191*(2), 773–784.

McFarland, C. T., Ly, L., Jeevan, A., Yamamoto, T., Weeks, B., Izzo, A., et al. (2010). BCG vaccination in the cotton rat (*Sigmodon hispidus*) infected by the pulmonary route with virulent *Mycobacterium tuberculosis*. *Tuberculosis (Edinburgh, Scotland), 90*(4), 262–267.

McMurray, D. N. (2001). Disease model: Pulmonary tuberculosis. *Trends in Molecular Medicine, 7*(3), 135–137.

McMurray, D. N., Bartow, R. A., & Mintzer, C. L. (1989). Impact of protein malnutrition on exogenous reinfection with *Mycobacterium tuberculosis*. *Infection and Immunity, 57*(6), 1746–1749.

Mehra, S., Pahar, B., Dutta, N. K., Conerly, C. N., Philippi-Falkenstein, K., Alvarez, X., et al. (2010). Transcriptional reprogramming in nonhuman primate (rhesus macaque) tuberculosis granulomas. *PLoS One, 5*(8), e12266.

Mehra, S., Golden, N. A., Dutta, N. K., Midkiff, C. C., Alvarez, X., Doyle, L. A., et al. (2011). Reactivation of latent tuberculosis in rhesus macaques by coinfection with simian immunodeficiency virus. *Journal of Medical Primatology, 40*(4), 233–243.

Meijer, A. H., & Spaink, H. P. (2011). Host-pathogen interactions made transparent with the zebrafish model. *Current Drug Targets, 12*(7), 1000–1017.

Metcoff, J., Darling, D., et al. (1949). Nutritional status and infection response; electrophoretic, circulating plasma protein, hematologic, hematopoietic, and pathologic responses to *Mycobacterium tuberculosis* (H37RV) infection in the protein-deficient rat. *The Journal of Laboratory and Clinical Medicine, 34*(3), 335–357.

Mgode, G. F., Cox, C. L., Mwimanzi, S., & Mulder, C. (2018). Pediatric tuberculosis detection using trained African giant pouched rats. *Pediatric Research*. https://doi.org/10.1038/pr.2018.40.

Michael, M., Jr., Cummings, M. M., & Bloom, W. L. (1950). Course of experimental tuberculosis in the albino rat as influenced by cortisone. *Proceedings of the Society for Experimental Biology and Medicine, 75*(2), 613–616.

Mothe, B. R., Lindestam Arlehamn, C. S., Dow, C., Dillon, M. B. C., Wiseman, R. W., Bohn, P., et al. (2015). The TB-specific CD4(+) T cell immune repertoire in both cynomolgus and rhesus macaques largely overlap with humans. *Tuberculosis (Edinburgh, Scotland), 95*(6), 722–735.

Mulder, C., Mgode, G. F., Ellis, H., Valverde, E., Beyene, N., Cox, C., et al. (2017a). Accuracy of giant African pouched rats for diagnosing tuberculosis: Comparison with culture and Xpert((R)) MTB/RIF. *The International Journal of Tuberculosis and Lung Disease, 21*(11), 1127–1133.

Mulder, C., Mgode, G., & Reid, S. E. (2017b). Tuberculosis diagnostic technology: An African solution ... think rats. *African Journal of Laboratory Medicine, 6*(2), 420.

Murohashi, T., Seki, M., & Yoshida, K. (1954). Inoculation with BCG and human type tubercle bacilli H37Rv to golden hamster. *Kekkaku: Tuberculosis, 29*(7), 239–242, English abstract, 72–3.

Nedeltchev, G. G., Raghunand, T. R., Jassal, M. S., Lun, S., Cheng, Q. J., & Bishai, W. R. (2009). Extrapulmonary dissemination of *Mycobacterium bovis* but not *Mycobacterium tuberculosis* in a bronchoscopic rabbit model of cavitary tuberculosis. *Infection and Immunity, 77*(2), 598–603.

North, R. J., & Jung, Y. J. (2004). Immunity to tuberculosis. *Annual Review of Immunology, 22*, 599–623.

Nuermberger, E. L. (2017). Preclinical efficacy testing of new drug candidates. *Microbiology Spectrum, 5*(3). https://doi.org/10.1128/microbiolspec.TBTB2-0034-2017.

Nusbaum, R. J., Calderon, V. E., Huante, M. B., Sutjita, P., Vijayakumar, S., Lancaster, K. L., et al. (2016). Pulmonary tuberculosis in humanized mice infected with HIV-1. *Scientific Reports, 6*, 21522.

Okada, M. (2006). Novel vaccines against *M. tuberculosis*. *Kekkaku. Tuberculosis, 81*(12), 745–751.

Oksanen, K. E., Halfpenny, N. J., Sherwood, E., Harjula, S. K., Hammaren, M. M., Ahava, M. J., et al. (2013). An adult zebrafish model for preclinical tuberculosis vaccine development. *Vaccine, 31*(45), 5202–5209.

Orme, I. M. (2003). The mouse as a useful model of tuberculosis. *Tuberculosis (Edinburgh, Scotland), 83*(1–3), 112–115.

Orme, I. M. (2005). Mouse and guinea pig models for testing new tuberculosis vaccines. *Tuberculosis (Edinburgh, Scotland), 85*(1–2), 13–17.

Orme, I. M. (2011). Development of new vaccines and drugs for TB: Limitations and potential strategic errors. *Future Microbiology, 6*(2), 161–177.

Padilha, E. C., Pires, R. V., Filho, M. A., de Pontes Machado, D. V., Baldan, H. M., Davanco, M. G., et al. (2012). Pharmacokinetic and safety evaluation of the use of ciprofloxacin on an isoniazid-rifampicin regimen in rabbits. *Biopharmaceutics & Drug Disposition, 33*(9), 501–509.

Pagan, A. J., Yang, C. T., Cameron, J., Swaim, L. E., Ellett, F., Lieschke, G. J., et al. (2015). Myeloid growth factors promote resistance to mycobacterial infection by curtailing granuloma necrosis through macrophage replenishment. *Cell Host & Microbe, 18*(1), 15–26.

Parikka, M., Hammaren, M. M., Harjula, S. K., Halfpenny, N. J., Oksanen, K. E., Lahtinen, M. J., et al. (2012). *Mycobacterium marinum* causes a latent infection that can be reactivated by gamma irradiation in adult zebrafish. *PLoS Pathogens, 8*(9), e1002944.

Pena, J. C., & Ho, W. Z. (2015). Monkey models of tuberculosis: Lessons learned. *Infection and Immunity, 83*(3), 852–862.

Phillips, B. L., Gautam, U. S., Bucsan, A. N., Foreman, T. W., Golden, N. A., Niu, T., et al. (2017). LAG-3 potentiates the survival of *Mycobacterium tuberculosis* in host phagocytes by modulating mitochondrial signaling in an in-vitro granuloma model. *PLoS One, 12*(9), e0180413.

Poling, A., Mahoney, A., Beyene, N., Mgode, G., Weetjens, B., Cox, C., et al. (2015). Using giant African pouched rats to detect human tuberculosis: A review. *The Pan African Medical Journal, 21*, 333.

Prunescu, C. C., Prunescu, P., & Scripcariu, D. (1979). Metchnikoff-Schaumann bodies in experimental Yersin's type tuberculosis induced with *Mycobacterium avium* in hamster. *Morphology and Embryology (Bucur), 25*(2), 171–174.

Rahman, S., Gudetta, B., Fink, J., Granath, A., Ashenafi, S., Aseffa, A., et al. (2009). Compartmentalization of immune responses in human tuberculosis: Few CD8+ effector T cells but elevated levels of FoxP3+ regulatory t cells in the granulomatous lesions. *The American Journal of Pathology, 174*(6), 2211–2224.

Ramakrishnan, L. (2013). The zebrafish guide to tuberculosis immunity and treatment. *Cold Spring Harbor Symposia on Quantitative Biology, 78*, 179–192.

Ramakrishnan, U., Grant, F., Goldenberg, T., Zongrone, A., & Martorell, R. (2012). Effect of women's nutrition before and during early pregnancy on maternal and infant outcomes: A systematic review. *Paediatric and Perinatal Epidemiology, 26*(Suppl 1), 285–301.

Ramos, L., Obregon-Henao, A., Henao-Tamayo, M., Bowen, R., Lunney, J. K., & Gonzalez-Juarrero, M. (2017). The minipig as an animal model to study Mycobacterium tuberculosis infection and natural transmission. *Tuberculosis (Edinburgh, Scotland), 106*, 91–98.

Ratcliffe, H. L., & Palladino, V. S. (1953). Tuberculosis induced by droplet nuclei infection; initial homogeneous response of small mammals (rats, mice, guinea pigs, and hamsters) to human and to bovine bacilli, and the rate and pattern of tubercle development. *The Journal of Experimental Medicine, 97*(1), 61–68.

Rawal, T., Parmar, R., Tyagi, R. K., & Butani, S. (2017). Rifampicin loaded chitosan nanoparticle dry powder presents an improved therapeutic approach for alveolar tuberculosis. *Colloids and Surfaces B: Biointerfaces, 154*, 321–330.

Rubin, E. J. (2009). The granuloma in tuberculosis--friend or foe? *The New England Journal of Medicine, 360*(23), 2471–2473.

Ryzewska, A. (1969). Influence of the composition of Freund's adjuvant, strain and sex of animals on the course of adjuvant--induced polyarthritis in rats. *Reumatologia, 7*(3), 195–206.

Schmidt, L. H. (1966). Studies on the antituberculous activity of ethambutol in monkeys. *Annals of the New York Academy of Sciences, 135*(2), 747–758.

Seo, H., Al Mahmud, H., Kim, S., Islam, M. I., Lee, K. I., Gil, Y. S., et al. (2018). Acute, sub-chronic oral toxicity, toxicokinetics, and genotoxicity studies of DFC-2, an antitubercular drug candidate. *Regulatory Toxicology and Pharmacology, 95*, 91–101.

Sharma, R., Kaur, R., Mukesh, M., & Sharma, V. L. (2018). Assessment of hepatotoxicity of first-line anti-tuberculosis drugs on Wistar rats. *Naunyn-Schmiedeberg's Archives of Pharmacology, 391*(1), 83–93.

Sharpe, S. A., Eschelbach, E., Basaraba, R. J., Gleeson, F., Hall, G. A., McIntyre, A., et al. (2009). Determination of lesion volume by MRI and stereology in a macaque model of tuberculosis. *Tuberculosis (Edinburgh, Scotland), 89*(6), 405–416.

Sharpe, S. A., McShane, H., Dennis, M. J., Basaraba, R. J., Gleeson, F., Hall, G., et al. (2010). Establishment of an aerosol challenge model of tuberculosis in rhesus macaques and an evaluation of endpoints for vaccine testing. *Clinical and Vaccine Immunology: CVI, 17*(8), 1170–1182.

Sharpe, S., White, A., Gleeson, F., McIntyre, A., Smyth, D., Clark, S., et al. (2016). Ultra low dose aerosol challenge with *Mycobacterium tuberculosis* leads to divergent outcomes in rhesus and cynomolgus macaques. *Tuberculosis (Edinburgh, Scotland), 96*, 1–12.

Shen, Y., Shen, L., Sehgal, P., Zhou, D., Simon, M., Miller, M., et al. (2001). Antiretroviral agents restore *Mycobacterium*-specific T-cell immune responses and facilitate controlling a fatal tuberculosis-like disease in Macaques coinfected with simian immunodeficiency virus and *Mycobacterium bovis* BCG. *Journal of Virology, 75*(18), 8690–8696.

Shen, Y., Zhou, D., Qiu, L., Lai, X., Simon, M., Shen, L., et al. (2002). Adaptive immune response of Vgamma2Vdelta2+ T cells during mycobacterial infections. *Science (New York, NY), 295*(5563), 2255–2258.

Shi, C., Shi, J., & Xu, Z. (2011). A review of murine models of latent tuberculosis infection. *Scandinavian Journal of Infectious Diseases, 43*(11–12), 848–856.

Shibata, M., Shimokawa, Y., Sasahara, K., Yoda, N., Sasabe, H., Suzuki, M., et al. (2017). Absorption, distribution and excretion of the anti-tuberculosis drug delamanid in rats: Extensive tissue distribution suggests potential therapeutic value for extrapulmonary tuberculosis. *Biopharmaceutics & Drug Disposition, 38*(4), 301–312.

Sibley, L., Dennis, M., Sarfas, C., White, A., Clark, S., Gleeson, F., et al. (2016). Route of delivery to the airway influences the distribution of pulmonary disease but not the outcome of *Mycobacterium tuberculosis* infection in rhesus macaques. *Tuberculosis (Edinburgh, Scotland), 96*, 141–149.

Smith, D. T., Bethune, N., & Wilson, J. L. (1930). Etiology of spontaneous pulmonary disease in the albino rat. *Journal of Bacteriology, 20*(5), 361–370.

Smith, D. W., Grover, A. A., & Nungester, W. J. (1953). Comparison of the immunizing properties of BCG, ultraviolet irradiated vaccines, and various lipid antigens in rats, mice and guinea pigs. *Medical Bulletin (Ann Arbor), 19*(5), 122–129.

Srivastava, S., & Gumbo, T. (2011). In vitro and in vivo modeling of tuberculosis drugs and its impact on optimization of doses and regimens. *Current Pharmaceutical Design, 17*(27), 2881–2888.

Srivastava, S., Grace, P. S., & Ernst, J. D. (2016). Antigen export reduces antigen presentation and limits T cell control of *M. tuberculosis*. *Cell Host & Microbe, 19*(1), 44–54.

Steenken, W., Jr., & Wagley, P. F. (1945). Comparison of the golden hamster with the guinea pig following inoculations of virulent tubercle bacilli. *Proceedings of the Society for Experimental Biology and Medicine, 60*, 255–257.

Stoop, E. J. M., Schipper, T., Rosendahl Huber, S. K., Nezhinsky, A. E., Verbeek, F. J., Gurcha, S. S., et al. (2011). Zebrafish embryo screen for mycobacterial genes involved in the initiation of granuloma formation reveals a newly identified ESX-1 component. *Disease Models & Mechanisms, 4*(4), 526–536.

Stoop, E. J., Mishra, A. K., Driessen, N. N., van Stempvoort, G., Bouchier, P., Verboom, T., et al. (2013). Mannan core branching of lipo(arabino)mannan is required for mycobacterial virulence in the context of innate immunity. *Cellular Microbiology, 15*(12), 2093–2108.

Subbian, S., Tsenova, L., Yang, G., O'Brien, P., Parsons, S., Peixoto, B., et al. (2011a). Chronic pulmonary cavitary tuberculosis in rabbits: A failed host immune response. *Open Biology, 1*(4), 110016.

Subbian, S., Tsenova, L., O'Brien, P., Yang, G., Koo, M. S., Peixoto, B., et al. (2011b). Phosphodiesterase-4 inhibition combined with isoniazid treatment of rabbits with pulmonary tuberculosis reduces macrophage activation and lung pathology. *The American Journal of Pathology, 179*(1), 289–301.

Subbian, S., Tsenova, L., O'Brien, P., Yang, G., Koo, M. S., Peixoto, B., et al. (2011c). Phosphodiesterase-4 inhibition alters gene expression and improves isoniazid-mediated clearance of *Mycobacterium tuberculosis* in rabbit lungs. *PLoS Pathogens, 7*(9), e1002262.

Subbian, S., Tsenova, L., O'Brien, P., Yang, G., Kushner, N. L., Parsons, S., et al. (2012). Spontaneous latency in a rabbit model of pulmonary tuberculosis. *The American Journal of Pathology, 181*(5), 1711–1724.

Sugawara, I., Yamada, H., & Mizuno, S. (2004). Pulmonary tuberculosis in spontaneously diabetic goto kakizaki rats. *The Tohoku Journal of Experimental Medicine, 204*(2), 135–145.

Sugawara, I., Yamada, H., & Mizuno, S. (2006). Nude rat (F344/N-rnu) tuberculosis. *Cellular Microbiology, 8*(4), 661–667.

Tobach, E., & Bloch, H. (1955). A study of the relationship between behavior and susceptibility to tuberculosis in rats and mice. *Bibliotheca Tuberculosea, 9*, 62–89.

Tobin, D. M., & Ramakrishnan, L. (2008). Comparative pathogenesis of *Mycobacterium marinum* and *Mycobacterium tuberculosis*. *Cellular Microbiology, 10*(5), 1027–1039.

Tobin, D. M., Vary, J. C., Jr., Ray, J. P., Walsh, G. S., Dunstan, S. J., Bang, N. D., et al. (2010). The lta4h locus modulates susceptibility to mycobacterial infection in zebrafish and humans. *Cell, 140*(5), 717–730.

Tobin, D. M., Roca, F. J., Oh, S. F., McFarland, R., Vickery, T. W., Ray, J. P., et al. (2012). Host genotype-specific therapies can optimize the inflammatory response to mycobacterial infections. *Cell, 148*(3), 434–446.

Tsara, V., Serasli, E., & Christaki, P. (2009). Problems in diagnosis and treatment of tuberculosis infection. *Hippokratia, 13*(1), 20–22.

Tsenova, L., Ellison, E., Harbacheuski, R., Moreira, A. L., Kurepina, N., Reed, M. B., et al. (2005). Virulence of selected *Mycobacterium tuberculosis* clinical isolates in the rabbit model of meningitis is dependent on phenolic glycolipid produced by the bacilli. *The Journal of Infectious Diseases, 192*(1), 98–106.

Tsenova, L., Harbacheuski, R., Ellison, E., Manca, C., & Kaplan, G. (2006). Aerosol exposure system for rabbits: Application to *M. Tuberculosis* infection. *Applied Biosafety, 11*(1), 7–14.

van der Woude, A. D., Stoop, E. J., Stiess, M., Wang, S., Ummels, R., van Stempvoort, G., et al. (2014). Analysis of SecA2-dependent substrates in *Mycobacterium marinum* identifies protein kinase G (PknG) as a virulence effector. *Cellular Microbiology, 16*(2), 280–295.

Verreck, F. A., Vervenne, R. A., Kondova, I., van Kralingen, K. W., Remarque, E. J., Braskamp, G., et al. (2009). MVA.85A boosting of BCG and an attenuated, phoP deficient *M. tuberculosis* vaccine both show protective efficacy against tuberculosis in rhesus macaques. *PLoS One, 4*(4), e5264.

Vervenne, R. A. W., Jones, S. L., van Soolingen, D., van der Laan, T., Andersen, P., Heidt, P. J., et al. (2004). TB diagnosis in non-human primates: Comparison of two interferon-γ assays and the skin test for identification of *Mycobacterium tuberculosis* infection. *Veterinary Immunology and Immunopathology, 100*(1), 61–71.

Via, L. E., Lin, P. L., Ray, S. M., Carrillo, J., Allen, S. S., Eum, S. Y., et al. (2008). Tuberculous granulomas are hypoxic in guinea pigs, rabbits, and nonhuman primates. *Infection and Immunity, 76*(6), 2333–2340.

Via, L. E., Weiner, D. M., Schimel, D., Lin, P. L., Dayao, E., Tankersley, S. L., et al. (2013). Differential virulence and disease progression following Mycobacterium tuberculosis complex infection of the common marmoset (*Callithrix jacchus*). *Infection and Immunity, 81*(8), 2909–2919.

Via, L. E., England, K., Weiner, D. M., Schimel, D., Zimmerman, M. D., Dayao, E., et al. (2015). A sterilizing tuberculosis treatment regimen is associated with faster clearance of bacteria in cavitary lesions in marmosets. *Antimicrobial Agents and Chemotherapy, 59*(7), 4181–4189.

Volkman, H. E., Clay, H., Beery, D., Chang, J. C. W., Sherman, D. R., & Ramakrishnan, L. (2004). Tuberculous granuloma formation is enhanced by a *Mycobacterium* virulence determinant. *PLoS Biology, 2*(11), e367.

Volkman, H. E., Pozos, T. C., Zheng, J., Davis, J. M., Rawls, J. F., & Ramakrishnan, L. (2010). Tuberculous granuloma induction via interaction of a bacterial secreted protein with host epithelium. *Science (New York, NY), 327*(5964), 466–469.

Wang, V. F., & Meng, C. H. (1951). The use of the Chinese hamsters (Cricetulus griseus) in the study of *Mycobacterium tuberculosis*. I. Comparison between the cultural method and animal inoculation for the primary isolation of tubercle bacilli. *Chinese Medical Journal, 69*(1–2), 80–85.

Wang, L., Zhao, J., Zhang, R., Mi, L., Shen, X., Zhou, N., et al. (2018). Drug-drug interactions between PA-824 and Darunavir based on pharmacokinetics inrRats by LC-MS-MS. *Journal of Chromatographic Science, 56*(4), 327–335.

Watkins, S. C., Maniar, S., Mosher, M., Roman, B. L., Tsang, M., & St Croix, C. M. (2012). High resolution imaging of vascular function in zebrafish. *PLoS One, 7*(8), e44018.

WHO. (2017). *Global tuberculosis report*. Geneva: World Health Organization.

Wolf, A. J., Linas, B., Trevejo-Nunez, G. J., Kincaid, E., Tamura, T., Takatsu, K., et al. (2007). *Mycobacterium tuberculosis* infects dendritic cells with high frequency and impairs their function in vivo. *Journal of Immunology (Baltimore, MD: 1950), 179*(4), 2509–2519.

Wong, S. C., Puaux, A. L., Chittezhath, M., Shalova, I., Kajiji, T. S., Wang, X., et al. (2010). Macrophage polarization to a unique phenotype driven by B cells. *European Journal of Immunology, 40*(8), 2296–2307.

Yang, C. T., Cambier, C. J., Davis, J. M., Hall, C. J., Crosier, P. S., & Ramakrishnan, L. (2012). Neutrophils exert protection in the early tuberculous granuloma by oxidative killing of *Mycobacteria* phagocytosed from infected macrophages. *Cell Host & Microbe, 12*(3), 301–312.

Yang, X., Wedajo, W., Yamada, Y., Dahlroth, S. L., Neo, J. J., Dick, T., et al. (2018). 1,3,5-triazaspiro[5.5]undeca-2,4-dienes as selective *Mycobacterium tuberculosis* dihydrofolate reductase inhibitors with potent whole cell activity. *European Journal of Medicinal Chemistry, 144*, 262–276.

Zhai, Q. Q., Pang, J., Li, G. Q., Li, C. R., Wang, Y. C., Yu, L. Y., et al. (2017). Preclinical pharmacokinetic analysis of (E)-Methyl-4-aryl-4-oxabut-2-enoate, a noval Ser/Thr protein kinase B inhibitor, in rats. *Acta Poloniae Pharmaceutica, 74*(1), 299–307.

Zhan, L., Tang, J., Sun, M., & Qin, C. (2017). Animal models for tuberculosis in translational and precision medicine. *Frontiers in Microbiology, 8*, 717.

Novel Antimycobacterial Drugs and Host-Directed Therapies for Tuberculosis

Garrett Teskey, Caleb Cato, Jennifer Hernandez, Preet Kaur, Jeff Koury, Mariana Lucero, Andrew Tran, and Vishwanath Venketaraman

Introduction

Tuberculosis is a venerable scourge that can be dated back to the ancient Egyptian era. Despite being the oldest documented infectious disease, its prevalence still remains remarkably high (Shepherd and Chapman 2016). In 2015 alone, 10.4 million new cases of TB were documented, and 1.8 million deaths (Shepherd and Chapman 2016). Accordingly, *M. tb* is the leading infectious cause of death worldwide (World Health Organization 2016a). This is due to the fact that *Mycobacterium tuberculosis* has a variety of cellular characteristics which allow it to evade the immune system. Upon initial infection, resident macrophages of the lungs initiate innate immune responses by generating cytokines, inflammasome, antimicrobial proteins, and reactive oxidative species (ROS), among other host responses (Van Crevel et al. 2002). Often, however, this innate immune response is insufficient in preventing infection, and thus, a T cell-mediated adaptive response is triggered. The T cell subtype, Th1, secretes interferon gamma (IFN-γ) as well as a variety of other cytokines to recruit/activate macrophages and other immune cells to trigger intracellular antimicrobial mechanisms (Munk and Emoto 1995). Classically, due to this host immune response, *M. tb* will then be sequestered and become dormant within an immune generated structure known as a granuloma, which is regarded as a latent

G. Teskey · C. Cato · J. Hernandez · P. Kaur · J. Koury · M. Lucero · A. Tran
Graduate College of Biomedical Sciences, Western University of Health Sciences, Pomona, CA, USA

V. Venketaraman (✉)
Graduate College of Biomedical Sciences, Western University of Health Sciences, Pomona, CA, USA

Department of Basic Medical Sciences, College of Osteopathic Medicine of the Pacific, Western University of Health Sciences, Pomona, CA, USA
e-mail: vvenketaraman@westernu.edu

© Springer Nature Switzerland AG 2018

99

V. Venketaraman (ed.), *Understanding the Host Immune Response Against Mycobacterium tuberculosis Infection*, https://doi.org/10.1007/978-3-319-97367-8_5

M. tb infection (LTBI). However, pulmonary debility and vast inflammation will typically result as a byproduct of this host-mediated immune response designed to liberate the lungs of the bacteria. Additionally, one of the hallmark traits of acquired immunodeficiency syndrome (AIDS), which is brought on by human immunodeficiency virus-1 (HIV-1) infection, is a greater susceptibility to opportunistic infections such as *M. tb* infection (Huang et al. 2014). Worldwide statistics done in 2016 suggest that roughly 36.7 million people are infected with HIV (World Health Organization 2016b). As many as 40–80% of people with AIDS are at risk of contracting *M. tb* among developing countries. According to a report in 2010, of the 34 million people living with HIV-1, 22.9 million live in the sub-Saharan Africa, a region where *M. tb* is endemic (Oni et al. 2013). Since the emergence of HIV-1 infection, extrapulmonary TB has become more common and appears in more than 50% of AIDS patients (Rieder et al. 1990). Opportunistic infections are normally not a strong concern among immunocompetent individuals; however, the excessive loss of CD4+ T helper cells in patients with advanced stages of HIV infection can lead to an impaired immune system which is unable to adequately respond to these infections (Kumarasamy et al. 2005; Vignesh et al. 2007). The current antibiotic treatment regimen which includes a combination of isoniazid, rifampin, ethambutol, and pyrazinamide has various weaknesses and limitations which can prolong disease resolution, including long treatment time, high toxicity, a relatively high rate of treatment failure, as well as possible resistance development. With multidrug-resistant (MDR) cases, less than half of all patients who enter treatment successfully complete it (Chung-Delgado et al. 2015). Therefore, many new treatment options are being explored to combat TB, and several recent developments in research and clinical trials have made significant advancements toward disease prevention.

New Antimycobacterial Drugs

The search for new or repurposed antimicrobial drugs to treat TB has been, like most pharmaceutical research, filled with early apparent successes that fail in later trials. Subsequently, new antimycobacterial compounds are highly sought after because they reduce the need for drug-susceptibility testing. However, as of 2016, only two new drugs were in confirmatory phase 3 trials for MDR *M. tb* (bedaquiline and delamanid) and only two new compounds were in phase 3 trials for drug-susceptible *M. tb* (sutezolid and pretomanid) (Pym et al. 2015; Gler et al. 2012; Skripconoka et al. 2012; Zhang et al. 2014; Louie et al. 2011; Wallis et al. 2014; Dawson et al. 2015). However, trials for sutezolid were ceased in 2016 due to its shared mechanism of efficacy (binding the 23s RNA present in *M. tb* and mitochondria) and toxicity, making dosing challenging. Additionally, major hepatic safety concerns have stalled pretomanid as well (Wallis et al. 2014; Dawson et al. 2015; Wallis et al. 2016). Two new compounds have recently entered phase 1 trials (Q203 and TBA-354), but unfortunately each appears to possess major flaws as well. Outside of these new drugs, most trials are reliant on repurposed or derivative antimicrobials (Wallis et al. 2016). Rifabutin, a derivative of rifampicin, appears to be active against MDR strains of *M. tb* containing an *rpoB* mutation at codon 516, which accounts for up to a third of South Africa's MDR TB; it also has minimal induction of CYP3A4, opening it up to combination treatments not available with rifampicin itself (Wallis et al. 2016; Sirgel et al. 2013; ElMaraachli et al. 2015; Davies et al. 2007). Clofazimine an antimicrobial/anti-inflammatory drug previously used in the treatment of leprosy appears promising, though still in early trial stages (Tang et al. 2015; Barry et al. 1960; Karat et al. 1970). Additionally, in vitro assays of carbapenems have shown promising potential such as faropenem and meropenem, as have sulfonamides (Anglaret et al. 1999; Walker et al. 2010; Hoffmann et al. 2014).

One of the greatest challenges in current TB treatment regimens, which has heavily contributed to the rise of drug resistance, is the long treatment duration and resulting noncompliance (Wallis et al. 2016). Because of this, a key focus of TB research has been on shorter drug regimens which limit the rate of patient relapse. While some trials have found that certain patient characteristics, such as a lack of cavitary disease upon diagnosis, allow for a shorter treatment duration, most focus on new regimens (Wallis et al. 2016). Trials on moxifloxacin and gatifloxacin appeared promising in early trials, but large phase 3 trials found that shortening treatment from 6 to 4 months increased relapse risk from less than 5% to 10% (Dawson et al. 2015; Gillespie et al. 2014; Jindani et al. 2014). High-dose rifampicin/rifapentine trials similarly found that a 4-month treatment increased relapse risk compared to 6-month regimens, this time up to 13% (Jindani et al. 2014; Dorman et al. 2015). Pretomanid doses of 100 and 200 mg were found in phase 2 trials to have predicted relapse rates of 16% and 10%, respectively, within 4-month treatment periods. Although the 200 mg dose only displayed a 10% relapse risk after 6 months of treatment in MDR patients, a promising result despite the mixed outcomes (Dawson et al. 2015). Consequently, pretomanid moved into phase 3 trials in 2015 but was quickly put on hold due to hepatic safety concerns (Wallis et al. 2016). Therefore, it appears that the antimicrobial drugs currently in clinical trials are not sufficient to profoundly ameliorate TB, but the momentum to discover new drugs for treatment as a whole appears to be growing, and host-directed therapies may be the superlative solution.

Host-Directed Therapies

Recognizing the potential significance host-directed therapies possess in response to *M. tb* infection is advancing as data continues to show favorable support. The use of new and repurposed drugs, biologics, and cell therapies to enhance host immune response by promoting autophagy, antimicrobial peptide production, and other macrophage effector mechanisms appears to be a promising area of research. To enhance antimicrobial mechanisms, a handful of drugs exist to induce autophagy, induce cathelicidins, or promote phagosome-lysosomal fusion. Autophagy is an intracellular process which degrades cytoplasmic material by shuttling it into the lysosome. Drugs such as rapamycin (an mTOR inhibitor) and Gefitinib (an epidermal growth factor receptor inhibitor) are a means to promote autophagy of ubiquitinylated *M. tb* to the lysosome (Ravikumar et al. 2004). Histone deacetylase inhibitors have been shown to epigenetically modify and promote cathelicidin expression. Cathelicidin is an antimicrobial protein which likewise promotes autophagy (Liu et al. 2006). Additionally, protein kinase (PK) inhibitors have also been repurposed to inhibit infection, specifically through increased acidification and maturation of the phagosome. Imatinib, developed by Novartis, is a PK inhibitor originally packaged for treating chromic myeloid leukemia (CML) but has recently been shown to reduce intracellular *M. tb* among mice cohorts (Bruns et al. 2012). Similarly, the diabetes drug metformin, a potential autophagy inducer, has been shown to reduce *M. tb* colony-forming units in vitro. One study found that diabetics treated with metformin who were concurrently suffering from active TB were significantly less likely to possess cavitary disease upon diagnosis nor die during their first year of diagnosis (Singhal et al. 2014).

Interestingly, intracellular protozoan parasites constitute a novel niche in the realm of host-directed therapies, capable of augmenting macrophage effector mechanisms against *M. tb*. The innate immune system has developed distinct strategies for detecting the cell markers present on eukaryotic pathogens (Yarovinsky 2014). However, information regarding the mechanisms by which protozoan parasites induce an innate immune response is only recently emerging (Debierre-Grockiego et al. 2007). Recent data suggests *Toxoplasma gondii*'s dense granule antigen 7 (GRA7) is capable of inducing an innate immune response among macrophages harboring a *M. tb* infection (Yang 2017; Koh et al. 2017). *T. gondii* is an apicomplexan protozoan parasite characterized by the formation of a parasitophorous vacuole (PV) upon host cell invasion (Schwab et al. 1994; Mercier et al. 2005). The function of this membrane-bounded vesicle is to protect the developing intracellular parasite from destructive phagolysosomes by preventing acidification of the internal compartment in which the parasite resides (Schwab et al. 1994; Mercier et al. 2005). Dense granules are one of three specialized secretory organelles involved in the formation of the PV membrane which are specific to apicomplexan parasites (Mercier et al. 2005). Dense granule antigens have shown promising potential as vaccine candidates for infectious diseases, most notably GRA7 (Jung et al. 2004). Koh et al. demonstrated that GRA7 interacts with signaling molecules involved in the antimicrobial response of the innate immune system (Koh et al. 2017). GRA7 was shown to be activated by phosphorylation via protein kinase C-α (PKC-α), which is a key regulator of macrophage effector mechanisms (Koh et al. 2017). Additionally, a phosphomimetic GRA7 mutant was capable of interacting with host antimicrobial response proteins in PKCα deficient cells both in vitro and in vivo (Koh et al. 2017). This finding is significant given that the downregulation of PKC-α in macrophages by *M. tb* has been shown to promote its survival by attenuating antimicrobial defense signaling pathways (Chaurasiya and Srivastava 2009). Most importantly, phosphorylation of GRA7 by PKCα facilitated GRA7 binding to inflammasome adaptor protein ASC (apoptosis-associated speck-like protein containing a carboxy-terminal CARD) and PLD1 (phospholipase D-1) which mediates phagolysosome biogenesis (Koh et al. 2017). Given that *M. tb* inhibits inflammasome activation and IL-1β production as well as phagolysosome maturation and biogenesis (Master et al. 2008; Deretic et al. 2006), GRA7's ability to activate the host antimicrobial defense mechanisms suppressed by *M. tb* suggests *T. gondii* antigens may contribute to antimicrobial defense against *M. tb*. For example, GRA7 induces the oligomerization of ASC (Yang 2017; Koh et al. 2017), an adaptor protein that connects Nod-like receptors (NLRs) to pro-caspase-1 facilitating NALP-containing inflammasome assembly and subsequent pro-IL-1β production (Master et al. 2008). Additionally, GRA7 binds to PLD1 initiating PLD1-dependent phagolysosome maturation and biogenesis (Yang 2017; Koh et al. 2017; Iyer et al. 2004). Koh et al. further substantiated these results in murine models, where GRA7 associated with ASC and PLD1 in vivo which resulted in reduced *M. tb* bacillary load in the lung, liver, and spleen, as well as a reduction in the size of granulomatous lesion formation in the lung of GRA7-vector-treated mice (Koh et al. 2017). These results indicate that *T. gondii*-induced, innate immune responses may provide a novel therapeutic strategy for the eradication of *M. tb* infection. However, before GRA7 can be seriously considered as a novel host-directed therapy, these results must be substantiated by additional preclinical studies and clinical trials. Therefore, it remains to be seen if GRA7 or protozoan antigens in general can constitute a viable strategy for host-directed therapies against *M. tb*.

For decades, high doses of vitamin D were commonly used to treat TB during the pre-antibiotic era. The prophylactic powers of vitamin D have often been thought to aid innate immune defenses against intracellular pathogens, however, in regard to TB the relationship is rather complex (Wilkinson et al. 2000). Patients with active TB often demonstrate a positive correlation with vitamin D insufficiency (VDI); however, there is no clear evidence that the reduction in vitamin D is related to the disease (Orkin et al. 2014). Vitamin D has many different roles within our bodies, and the majority of vitamin D we use comes from the ultraviolet β-induced cleavage of 7-dehydrocholesterol in skin cells which is then converted to calcidiol (25-hydroxy vitamin D3) in the liver, and then undergoes α-hydroxylation in the kidneys to produce calcitriol (1, 25-hydroxy vitamin D3), the final active form (Coussens et al. 2014). High concentrations of calcitriol when added to *M. tb*-infected blood mononuclear cell cultures have been shown to inhibit the production of interferon-γ, TNF, and IL-12 (Martineau et al. 2007). Although numerous clinical studies have tested the effects of vitamin D against *M. tb* infection, many of these studies fail to show any significant efficacy against *M. tb* infection (Wallis and Zumla 2016). However, the findings reported by Mily et al. indicate that vitamin D significantly reduced the proportion of positive cultures after 8 weeks of treatment (Mily et al. 2015). Additionally, Wallis et al. postulated that if the same treatment was given for 4 months, the relapse rate would be as low as 6%, and there should only be a 15% chance of the relapse rate exceeding 10% (Wallis and Zumla 2016). Taken together these findings support the prospective use of adjunctive host-directed therapies to increase antimicrobial activation mechanisms.

Host-Directed Therapies That Reduce Inflammation

The other categories of HDTs are involved in inhibiting mechanisms which cause long-term tissue damage such as lung inflammation or reducing matrix destruction, due to a prolonged host immune response. However, anti-inflammatory treatment still remains controversial in regard to *M. tb* infection due to the fact that granuloma initiation generally requires an inflammatory response mediated by suitable cell signaling. Of the variety of methods to reduce TB inflammation, some that have gone into preclinical/clinical trials include corticosteroids, TNF-α inhibitors, and COX inhibitors. Corticosteroids have been shown to reduce the signs and symptoms of TB and potentially reduce mortality (Dooley et al. 1997; Critchley et al. 2013). In a clinical trial (NCT00057421), the corticosteroid prednisone was administered to 187 HIV-TB patients. The patients who took prednisone showed an explicit reduction in positive sputum cultures when compared to the placebo. TNF-α blockers are commonly administered for autoimmune disorders, to suppress the inflammatory events (Sethi et al. 2009). Thus, TNF-α blocking monoclonal antibodies show great promise in reducing adverse inflammation from *M. tb*. However, unfortunately they have a propensity to reactivate latent tuberculosis at a rate of 21% (Wallis et al. 2004). COX inhibitors, such as ibuprofen, have been shown to prolong survival in mice, potentially due to neutrophil reduction at the site of inflammation (Vilaplana et al. 2013). However, no formal human trial studies have yet been published for treating active TB with COX inhibitors.

Additionally, doxycycline and CC-11050 have been proposed for further investigation as TB therapeutics due to their potential to inhibit lung damage during the course of the disease (Ong et al. 2015; Subbian et al. 2011a). Doxycycline nonspecifically inhibits matrix metalloproteinases, which animal models have shown to be an important factor in TB lung pathology (Ong et al. 2015). CC-11050, previously approved for anti-inflammatory diseases, has been demonstrated to reduce the number and size of lung granulomas in both mice and rabbits, as well as accelerate isoniazid induced bacillary clearance (Subbian et al. 2011a; Kavanaugh et al. 2014; Paul et al. 2015; Subbian et al. 2011b; Koo et al. 2011).

A recent study on TB by Judy et al. involving HIV positive individuals discovered that they possessed diminished levels of the biological antioxidant glutathione (GSH) (Ly et al. 2015). They subsequently established the relationship between GSH deficiency, HIV disease progression, and increased susceptibility to *M. tb* infection. GSH is a tripeptide antioxidant involved in maintaining redox homeostasis, and is essential for many cellular functions such as protein synthesis, apoptosis, transmembrane transport, and enzyme catalysis (Ballatori et al. 2009). Previous work from Dr. Venketaraman's laboratory demonstrated that decreased levels of GSH are also accompanied by an impaired immune response against *M. tb* infection (Allen et al. 2015). Additionally, GSH has been shown to have direct antimycobacterial activity and functions as an effector molecule in the immune defense against *M. tb* infection. GSH has been shown to alter cytokine expression and enhance the activity of natural killer cells to inhibit *M. tb* growth inside macrophages (Guerra et al. 2012). Furthermore, GSH can activate CD4+ T-cells which provide additional control over the *M. tb* infection (Guerra et al. 2011). The lab has demonstrated that the total and reduced forms of GSH are significantly decreased among macrophages, NK cells, and T cells derived from the peripheral blood of HIV-1 infected individuals (Guerra et al. 2011; Morris et al. 2012). Therefore, the researchers conducted a clinical trial with the hypothesis that supplementing HIV positive individuals with GSH will lead to an increase in the levels of beneficial Th1 cytokines as well as a reduction in reactive oxygen species. This ultimately translates into enhanced *M. tb* control, as the oxidative stress and redox imbalance that arises from HIV-1 infection can result in inappropriate immune responses. Thus maintaining redox homeostasis allows for protective host immune responses against intracellular infections such as *M. tb* (Venketaraman et al. 2005). The researchers established that after GSH supplementation, the HIV+ individuals had a marked decrease in their plasma levels of TGF-β which corresponded with a significant increase in their GSH levels as well (Ly et al. 2015). These individuals also displayed a decrease in IL-6 and ROS markers after GSH supplementation compared to their initial levels at the start of the study (Ly et al. 2015). Notably, the results of this experiment also revealed a prominent decrease in the *M. tb* colony forming units among the HIV+ participants who received GSH supplementation, whereas the cytokine and GSH levels of the patients receiving the placebo showed no significant difference from their initial visit (Ly et al. 2015). These studies establish that GSH supplementation can lead to a decrease in oxidative stress, beneficial cytokines modulation, and most importantly a decrease in *M. tb* bioburden.

Biomarkers

Research on TB biomarkers has become extremely important in the fight against *M. tb* infection. More accurate biomarkers can lead to faster drug trials, more successful treatment, and less time wasted when treating with ineffective drugs. The majority of current TB biomarker research encompasses sputum cultures, PET scans, or gene expression profiles (Wallis et al. 2016). Sputum-culture status at 2-months has a strong positive association with treatment success or failure, allowing for faster patient turn-around when on ineffective drug regimens, and provides new methods for predicting risk of relapse during drug trials. Another emerging technique used for assessing TB is PET scan in combination with CT imaging which provides a noninvasive testing method for disease activity, response to therapy, and early relapse risk. Finally, research into the genetic, epigenetic, and proteomic signatures of *M. tb* have identified specific gene signatures predicting the development of active TB disease among patients with latent TB.

Conclusion

The US Presidential Executive Order Combating Antibiotic-Resistant Bacteria has created a new framework for clinical and nonclinical trials (Obama 2014). Thus, a new approval process has been set in motion, one which is ideal for research and accelerated approval of MDR TB. Auxiliary development could conceivably even replace the requirement for large-scale phase 3 trials with smaller studies and enhance post-licensing outcome reporting. Increased approval rates as well as a more efficient and realistic regulatory mechanism for TB drugs and therapeutics could ideally have a drastic and profound effect on the incidence of TB worldwide. Although the current antimicrobial drugs in clinical trials do not appear to drastically power this progression, there are genuine prospects in the realm of host-directed therapies. Both host-directed therapies which increase antimicrobial activation and which reduce harmful inflammation, as we have discussed previously, present explicit potentiality to alleviate the destructive capacity of a *M. tb* infection. Nevertheless, more research is undoubtedly required in these areas for this aspiration to come to fruition.

References

Allen, M., et al. (2015). Mechanisms of control of *Mycobacterium tuberculosis* by NK cells: *Role of Glutathione. Frontiers in Immunology, 6*, 508.

Anglaret, X., Chêne, G., Attia, A., the Cotrimo-CI Study Group, et al. (1999). Early chemoprophylaxis with trimethoprim-sulphamethoxazole for HIV-1-infected adults in Abidjan, Côte d'Ivoire: A randomised trial. *Lancet, 353*, 1463–1468.

Ballatori, N., et al. (2009). Glutathione dysregulation and the etiology and progression of human diseases. *Biological Chemistry, 390*(3), 191–214.

Barry, V. C., Buggle, K., Byrne, J., Conalty, M. L., & Winder, F. (1960). Absorption, distribution and retention of the riminocompounds in the experimental animal. *Irish Journal of Medical Science, 416*, 345–352.

Bruns, H., et al. (2012). Abelson tyrosine kinase controls phagosomal acidification required for killing of Mycobacterium tuberculosis in human macrophages. *Journal of Immunology, 189*(8), 4069–4078.

Chaurasiya, S. K., & Srivastava, K. K. (2009). Downregulation of protein kinase C-alpha enhances intracellular survival of Mycobacteria: Role of PknG. *BMC Microbiology, 9*, 271.

Chung-Delgado, K., Guillen-Bravo, S., Revilla-Montag, A., & Bernabe-Ortiz, A. (2015). Mortality among MDR-TB cases: Comparison with drug-susceptible tuberculosis and associated factors. *PLoS One, 10*(3), e0119332.

Coussens, A. K., Martineau, A. R., & Wilkinson, R. J. (2014). Anti-inflammatory and antimicrobial actions of vitamin D in combating TB/HIV. *Scientifica (Cairo), 2014*, 903680.

Critchley, J. A., Young, F., Orton, L., & Garner, P. (2013). Corticosteroids for prevention of mortality in people with tuberculosis: A systematic review and meta-analysis. *The Lancet Infectious Diseases, 13*, 223–237.

Davies, G., Cerri, S., & Richeldi, L. (2007). Rifabutin for treating pulmonary tuberculosis. *Cochrane Database of Systematic Reviews, 4*, CD005159.

Dawson, R., Diacon, A. H., Everitt, D., van Niekerk, C., Donald, P. R., Burger, D. A., et al. (2015). Efficiency and safety of the combination of moxifloxacin, pretomanid (PA-824), and pyrazinamide during the first 8 weeks of antituberculosis treatment: a phase 2b, open-label, partly randomised trial in patients with drug-susceptible or drug-resistant pulmonary tuberculosis. *Lancet, 385*, 1738–1747.

Debierre-Grockiego, F., et al. (2007). Activation of TLR2 and TLR4 by glycosylphosphatidylinositols derived from Toxoplasma gondii. *Journal of Immunology, 179*(2), 1129–1137.

Deretic, V., et al. (2006). Mycobacterium tuberculosis inhibition of phagolysosome biogenesis and autophagy as a host defence mechanism. *Cellular Microbiology, 8*(5), 719–727.

Dooley, D. P., Carpenter, J. L., & Rademacher, S. (1997). Adjunctive corticosteroid therapy for tuberculosis: A critical reappraisal of the literature. *Clinical Infectious Diseases, 25*, 872–887.

Dorman, S. E., Savic, R. M., Goldberg, S., et al. (2015). Daily rifapentine for treatment of pulmonary tuberculosis. A randomized, dose-ranging trial. *American Journal of Respiratory and Critical Care Medicine, 191*, 333–343.

ElMaraachli, W., Slater, M., Berrada, Z. L., et al. (2015). Predicting differential rifamycin resistance in clinical *Mycobacterium tuberculosis* isolates by specific *rpo*B mutations. *The International Journal of Tuberculosis and Lung Disease, 19*, 1222–1226.

Gillespie, S. H., Crook, A. M., McHugh, T. D., et al. (2014). Four-month moxifloxacin-based regimens for drug-sensitive tuberculosis. *The New England Journal of Medicine, 371*, 1577–1587.

Gler, M. T., Skripconoka, V., Sanchez-Garavito, E., et al. (2012). Delamanid for multidrug-resistant pulmonary tuberculosis. *The New England Journal of Medicine, 366*, 2151–2160.

Guerra, C., et al. (2011). Glutathione and adaptive immune responses against *Mycobacterium tuberculosis* infection in healthy and HIV infected individuals. *PLoS One, 6*(12), e28378.

Guerra, C., et al. (2012). *Control of Mycobacterium tuberculosis* growth by activated natural killer cells. *Clinical and Experimental Immunology, 168*(1), 142–152.

Hoffmann, C. J., Chaisson, R. E., & Martinson, N. A. (2014). Cotrimoxazole prophylaxis and tuberculosis risk among people living with HIV. *PLoS One, 9*, e83750.

Huang, C. C., Tchetgen, E. T., Becerra, M. C., Cohen, T., Hughes, K. C., Zhang, Z., Calderon, R., Yataco, R., Contreras, C., Galea, J., Lecca, L., & Murray, M. (2014). The effect of HIV-related immunosuppression on the risk of tuberculosis transmission to household contacts. *Clinical Infectious Diseases, 58*(6), 765–774.

Iyer, S. S., et al. (2004). Phospholipases D1 and D2 coordinately regulate macrophage phagocytosis. *Journal of Immunology, 173*(4), 2615–2623.

Jindani, A., Harrison, T. S., Nunn, A. J., et al. (2014). High-dose rifapentine with moxifloxacin for pulmonary tuberculosis. *The New England Journal of Medicine, 371*, 1599–1608.

Jung, C., Lee, C. Y., & Grigg, M. E. (2004). The SRS superfamily of Toxoplasma surface proteins. *International Journal for Parasitology, 34*(3), 285–296.

Karat, A. B., Jeevaratnam, A., Karat, S., & Rao, P. S. (1970). Double-blind controlled clinical trial of clofazimine in reactive phases of lepromatous leprosy. *British Medical Journal, 1*, 198–200.

Kavanaugh, A., Mease, P. J., Gomez-Reino, J. J., et al. (2014). Treatment of psoriatic arthritis in a phase 3 randomised, placebo-controlled trial with apremilast, an oral phosphodiesterase 4 inhibitor. *Annals of the Rheumatic Diseases, 73*, 1020–1026.

Koh, H. J., et al. (2017). *Toxoplasma gondii* GRA7-targeted ASC and PLD1 promote antibacterial host defense via PKCalpha. *PLoS Pathogens, 13*(1), e1006126.

Koo, M. S., Manca, C., Yang, G., et al. (2011). Phosphodiesterase 4 inhibition reduces innate immunity and improves isoniazid clearance of *Mycobacterium tuberculosis* in the lungs of infected mice. *PLoS One, 6*, e17091.

Kumarasamy, N., Vallabhaneni, S., Flanigan, T. P., Mayer, K. H., & Solomon, S. (2005). Clinical profile of HIV in India. *The Indian Journal of Medical Research, 121*, 377–394.

Liu, P. T., et al. (2006). Toll-like receptor triggering of a vitamin D-mediated human antimicrobial response. *Science, 311*(5768), 1770–1773.

Louie, A., Eichas, K., & Files, K., et al. (2011). *Activities of PNU-100480 (PNU 480) alone, PNU 480 plus its major metabolite PNU-101603 (PNU 1603) and PNU 480 plus PNU 1603 in combination with rifampin (RIF) against* Mycobacterium tuberculosis: *comparison with linezolid.* Interscience Conference on Antimicrobial Agents and Chemotherapy, Chicago, IL, 17–20 Sept 2011, pp. A1–1737.

Ly, J., Lagman, M., Saing, T., Singh, M. K., Tudela, E. V., Morris, D., & Venketaraman, V. (2015). Liposomal glutathione supplementation restores TH1 cytokine response to *Mycobacterium tuberculosis* infection in HIV-infected individuals. *Journal of Interferon & Cytokine Research, 35*(11), 875–887.

Martineau, A. R., Wilkinson, K. A., Newton, S. M., et al. (2007). IFN-gamma- and TNF- independent vitamin D-inducible human suppression of mycobacteria: The role of cathelicidin LL-37. *Journal of Immunology, 178*, 7190–7198.

Master, S. S., et al. (2008). Mycobacterium tuberculosis prevents inflammasome activation. *Cell Host & Microbe, 3*(4), 224–232.

Mercier, C., et al. (2005). Dense granules: Are they key organelles to help understand the parasitophorous vacuole of all apicomplexa parasites? *International Journal for Parasitology, 35*(8), 829–849.

Mily, A., Rekha, R. S., Kamal, S. M., et al. (2015). Significant effects of oral phenylbutyrate and vitamin D3 adjunctive therapy in pulmonary tuberculosis: A randomized controlled trial. *PLoS One, 10*, e0138340.

Morris, D., et al. (2012). Unveiling the mechanisms for decreased glutathione in individuals with HIV infection. *Clinical & Developmental Immunology, 2012*, 734125.

Munk, M. E., & Emoto, M. (1995). Functions of T-cell subsets and cytokines in mycobacterial infections. *The European Respiratory Journal. Supplement, 20*, 668s–675s.

Obama, B. (2014). *The Executive Order—combating antibiotic-resistant bacteria.* http://www.whitehouse.gov/the-press-office/2014/09/18/executive-order-combating-antibiotic-resistant-bacteria. Accessed 28 Dec 2015.

Ong, C. W., Elkington, P. T., Brilha, S., et al. (2015). Neutrophil-derived MMP-8 drives AMPK-dependent matrix destruction in human pulmonary tuberculosis. *PLoS Pathogens, 11*, e1004917.

Oni, T., Stoever, K., & Wilkinson, R. J. (2013). Tuberculosis, HIV, and type 2 diabetes mellitus: A neglected priority. *The Lancet Respiratory Medicine, 1*(5), 356–358.

Orkin, C., Wohl, D. A., Williams, A., & Deckx, H. (2014). Vitamin D deficiency in HIV: A shadow on long-term management? *AIDS Reviews, 16*, 59–74.

Paul, C., Cather, J., Gooderham, M., et al. (2015). Efficacy and safety of apremilast, an oral phosphodiesterase 4 inhibitor, in patients with moderate-to-severe plaque psoriasis over 52 weeks: A phase III, randomized controlled trial (ESTEEM 2). *The British Journal of Dermatology, 173*, 1387–1399.

Pym, A. S., Diacon, A. H., Tang, S. J., et al. (2015). Bedaquiline in the treatment of multidrug- and extensively drug-resistant tuberculosis. *The European Respiratory Journal, 47*, 564–574.

Ravikumar, B., et al. (2004). Inhibition of mTOR induces autophagy and reduces toxicity of polyglutamine expansions in fly and mouse models of Huntington disease. *Nature Genetics, 36*(6), 585–595.

Rieder, H. L., Snider, D. E., Jr., & Cauthen, G. M. (1990). Extrapulmonary tuberculosis in the United States. *The American Review of Respiratory Disease, 141*(2), 347–351.

Schwab, J. C., Beckers, C. J., & Joiner, K. A. (1994). The parasitophorous vacuole membrane surrounding intracellular Toxoplasma gondii functions as a molecular sieve. *Proceedings of the National Academy of Sciences of the United States of America, 91*(2), 509–513.

Sethi, G., Sung, B., Kunnumakkara, A. B., & Aggarwal, B. B. (2009). Targeting TNF for treatment of cancer and autoimmunity. *Advances in Experimental Medicine and Biology, 647*, 37–51. https://doi.org/10.1007/978-0-387-89520-8_3.

Shepherd, J. G., & Chapman, A. L. N. (2016). Assessment and management of active and latent TB. *Practitioner, 260*(1798), 21–24.

Singhal, A., Kumar, P., Hong, G. S., et al. (2014). Metformin as adjunct anti-tuberculosis therapy. *Science Translational Medicine, 6*, 263ra159.

Sirgel, F. A., Warren, R. M., Bottger, E. C., Klopper, M., & Victor, T. C. (2013). The rationale for using rifabutin in the treatment of MDR and XDR tuberculosis outbreaks. *PLoS One, 8*, e59414.

Skripconoka, V., Danilovits, M., Pehme, L., et al. (2012). Delamanid improves outcomes and reduces mortality for multidrug-resistant tuberculosis. *The European Respiratory Journal, 41*, 1393–1400.

Subbian, S., Tsenova, L., O'Brien, P., et al. (2011a). Phosphodiesterase-4 inhibition combined with isoniazid treatment of rabbits with pulmonary tuberculosis reduces macrophage activation and lung pathology. *The American Journal of Pathology, 179*, 289–301.

Subbian, S., Tsenova, L., O'Brien, P., et al. (2011b). Phosphodiesterase-4 inhibition alters gene expression and improves isoniazid-mediated clearance of *Mycobacterium tuberculosis* in rabbit lungs. *PLoS Pathogens, 7*, e1002262.

Tang, S., Yao, L., Hao, X., et al. (2015). Clofazimine for the treatment of multidrug-resistant tuberculosis: Prospective, multicenter, randomized controlled study in China. *Clinical Infectious Diseases, 60*, 1361–1367.

Van Crevel, R., Ottenhoff, T. H. M., & van der Meer, J. W. M. (2002). Innate immunity to Mycobacterium tuberculosis. *Clinical Microbiology Reviews, 15*(2), 294–309.

Venketaraman, V., et al. (2005). Glutathione and nitrosoglutathione in macrophage defense against *Mycobacterium tuberculosis*. *Infection and Immunity, 73*(3), 1886–1889.

Vignesh, R., Balakrishnan, P., Shankar, E. M., Murugavel, K. G., Hanas, S., Cecelia, A. J., Thyagarajan, S. P., Solomon, S., & Kumarasamy, N. (2007). High proportion of isosporiasis among HIV- infected patients with diarrhea in southern India. *The American Journal of Tropical Medicine and Hygiene, 77*(5), 823–824.

Vilaplana, C., et al. (2013). Ibuprofen therapy resulted in significantly decreased tissue bacillary loads and increased survival in a new murine experimental model of active tuberculosis. *The Journal of Infectious Diseases, 208*(2), 199–202.

Walker, A. S., Ford, D., Gilks, C. F., et al. (2010). Daily co-trimoxazole prophylaxis in severely immunosuppressed HIV-infected adults in Africa started on combination antiretroviral therapy: An observational analysis of the DART cohort. *Lancet, 375*, 1278–1286.

Wallis, R. S., & Zumla, A. (2016). Vitamin D as adjunctive host-directed therapy in tuberculosis: A systematic review. *Open Forum Infectious Diseases, 3*(3), ofw151.

Wallis, R. S., et al. (2004). Granulomatous infections due to tumor necrosis factor blockade: Correction. *Clinical Infectious Diseases, 39*(8), 1254–1255.

Wallis, R. S., Dawson, R., Friedrich, S. O., et al. (2014). Mycobactericidal activity of sutezolid (PNU-100480) in sputum (EBA) and blood (WBA) of patients with pulmonary tuberculosis. *PLoS One, 9*, e94462.

Wallis, R. S., Maeurer, M., Mwaba, P., Chakaya, J., Rustomjee, R., Migliori, G. B., Marais, B., Schito, M., Churchyard, G., Swaminathan, S., Hoelscher, M., & Zumla, A. (2016). Tuberculosis—advances in development of new drugs, treatment regimens,host-directed therapies, and biomarkers. *The Lancet Infectious Diseases, 16*(4), e34–e46.

Wilkinson, R. J., Llewelyn, M., Toossi, Z., et al. (2000). Influence of vitamin D deficiency and vitamin D receptor polymorphisms on tuberculosis among Gujarati Asians in West London: A case-control study. *Lancet, 355*, 618–621.

World Health Organization. (2016a). *Tuberculosis (TB)*. Available online: http://www.who.int/TB/en/. Accessed 7 Oct 2017.

World Health Organization. (2016b). *HIV*. Available online: http://www.who.int/mediacentre/factsheets/fs360/en/. Accessed 7 Oct 2017.

Yang, C. S. (2017). Advancing host-directed therapy for tuberculosis. *Microbial Cell, 4*(3), 105–107.

Yarovinsky, F. (2014). Innate immunity to Toxoplasma gondii infection. *Nature Reviews. Immunology, 14*(2), 109–121.

Zhang, M., Sala, C., Dhar, N., et al. (2014). In vitro and in vivo activities of three oxazolidinones against nonreplicating *Mycobacterium tuberculosis*. *Antimicrobial Agents and Chemotherapy, 58*, 3217–3223.

Cigarette Smoking and Increased Susceptibility to *Mycobacterium tuberculosis* Infection

John Brazil and Vishwanath Venketaraman

Introduction

Cigarette smoking (CS) and tuberculosis (TB) are notorious for their lethality and ubiquity in the developing world. TB is the most prevalent infectious disease in the world and cigarette smoking is the most common cause of preventable death worldwide (Connell and Venketaraman 2009; Smoking and Tobacco Use 2018; Samet 2018). The linkage between cigarette smoking and TB is a somewhat intuitive observation that was first recognized by the scientific community in 1918; however, the accumulation of evidence to substantiate this hypothesis has taken nearly a century (Webb 1918; Slama et al. 2018).

The World Health Organization estimates that as much as a quarter of the world's population is latently infected with *Mycobacterium tuberculosis* (*M. tb* – causative agent of TB). Only slightly less common is cigarette smoking, which is practiced by an estimated 20.7% of the world's population (World Health Organization 2017). Of these approximately 1.1 billion smokers, more than 6 million will die every year as a direct result of smoking tobacco with an additional 890,000 nonsmokers dying from secondhand smoke-related maladies (World Health Organization 2017).

In addition to the prevalence of these diseases, what is especially concerning is the crossover between the demographics of these groups and that they often coexist in the same social and geographic niches. Estimates have found that 80% of the world's smokers live in low-to middle-income countries which classify the same socioeconomic strata that 95% of TB fatalities occur (World Health Organization

J. Brazil
The Master's University, Santa Clarita, CA, USA

V. Venketaraman (✉)
Department of Basic Medical Sciences, College of Osteopathic Medicine of the Pacific,
Western University of Health Sciences, Pomona, CA, USA
e-mail: vvenketaraman@westernu.edu

© Springer Nature Switzerland AG 2018   111
V. Venketaraman (ed.), *Understanding the Host Immune Response Against*
Mycobacterium tuberculosis Infection, https://doi.org/10.1007/978-3-319-97367-8_6

2017). This is especially true in China and India (Lönnroth et al. 2018). WHO estimated 23% of TB cases are attributable to smoking in the 23 countries that account for 80% of the world's TB (WHO 2010; Surgeon General Report 2014).

It was only 20 years ago that public officials in the United States believed TB would cease to be a major public health concern (Owen et al. 2013). Nearly a half million cases of multidrug-resistant TB (MDR-TB) were documented in the last year alone (World Health Organization 2018a). This thinking has drastically changed in the recent past with the rise of AIDS and MDR-TB and has even caused some to refer to this latest crisis as the third epidemic of TB.

As has been well-documented previously, individuals with HIV infection and people with type 2 diabetes are increasingly susceptible to TB. This chapter will explore the relationship between the aggravating effects of cigarette smoke compromising the ability of the immune system to combat *M. tb* infection thereby putting otherwise healthy individuals at high risk for susceptibility to *M. tb* infection.

Cigarette Smoking and TB

Logical inference and a hundred years of investigation implicate CS with increased susceptibility to *M. tb* infection. That being said there are multiple confounding variables in the analysis of the effect of CS on a population's vulnerability to TB and only recently have enough comprehensive studies been performed to draw any conclusions. The Surgeon General's 50-year report on The Health Consequences of Smoking thoroughly reviewed the literature and made the following conclusions (Surgeon General Report 2014):

1. A causal relationship exists between smoking and an increased risk for susceptibility to *M. tb* infection.
2. Cigarette smoking has been linked to increased mortality due to TB.
3. The existing evidence implicates but is inadequate to confirm a causal relationship between smoking and the risk of TB recurrence.
4. The evidence is insufficient to conclude either the presence or absence of a causal relationship between active smoking and the risks for contracting *M. tb*.
5. The evidence is insufficient to conclude either the presence or absence of a causal relationship between exposure to secondhand smoke and the risk for acquiring *M. tb* infection.
6. The evidence is insufficient to conclude either the presence or absence of a causal relationship between exposure to secondhand smoke and the risks for developing active disease.

For our purposes we will discuss the first four of these points and go on to describe potential mechanisms of causation. For those where the evidence is inadequate to indicate a causal relationship, keep in mind that this does not exclude the possibility. Rather, this speaks to the difficulty in conducting and analyzing comprehensive studies that limit confounding variables and have a statistically significant sample size. For example, studies have been conducted on the effect of passive smoke on children's likelihood of developing TB disease and have found positive correlations as high as fivefold (Kuemmerer and Comstock 1967), but the SGR still found the evidence inadequate to confirm a causal relationship between secondhand smoke and TB. Therefore, in many cases evidence exists that implicates causation but is perhaps not satisfactory—as of yet—to make any definitive claims.

Cigarette Smoking and TB Disease

Substantial evidence has shown that a causative relationship exists between CS and active TB. Although confounding variables (alcohol use, exposure to TB, SES, etc.) are often present in the sample populations, there has been sufficient evidence subjected to statistical derivation which affirms a causative relationship between active TB and CS. One particularly significant study found a fourfold increase in risk of TB disease among active smokers, although other studies place a more conservative estimate of increased risk at twofold (Lin et al. 2009; Yu et al. 1988). The increase in risk of TB disease was more strongly correlated with the length of time a person smoked in comparison to the intensity of their smoking (Prasad et al. 2009). Interestingly enough, this trend was not true for children and at least one study found that the number of cigarettes children was exposed to directly relate to an increased risk for developing active TB disease (Kuemmerer and Comstock 1967). The majority of these studies were conducted internationally, but at least one conducted in the United States affirmed this same trend (Smith et al. 2018). The variety of locations and settings in which these studies have been conducted naturally eliminates many confounding variables and strengthens the collective findings.

One other point of interest is that this relationship between TB disease and CS has also been demonstrated in male victims of HIV (Bronner Murrison et al. 2016). This could be a particularly relevant point to mitigate the substantial risks to infection that HIV patients are already under.

Cigarette Smoking and Mortality Due to TB

Sufficient studies have confirmed an increased incidence of TB mortality associated with CS (Jha et al. 2008). Studies in China, Africa, Hong Kong, India, and Korea have all found a positive correlation that implicates CS with increased mortality (Jha et al. 2008; Liu et al. 1998; Lam et al. 2001; Jee et al. 2009; Gajalakshmi et al. 2003; Jha et al. 2008; Sitas et al. 2004). One of these studies that was performed in India found that as much as 38% of TB deaths were caused by CS (Jha et al. 2008). It was approximated that in India more than 140,000 TB deaths per year were due to CS, which accounted for more than 50% of TB deaths. A global WHO analysis of the burden of TB found that 80% of the global TB burden could be concentrated in 22 countries, and in those 22 countries 23% of the TB cases can be attributed to CS (WHO 2010). It is worth noting that the driving force of TB differs depending on the country in question. In China and India, a high proportion of TB cases can be linked to CS whereas in sub-Saharan Africa, HIV is the driving force (Lonnroth et al. 2010).

CS has also been shown to diminish the formation of granulomas and effector responses against *M. tb* within the granulomas which are crucial for two reasons (Owen et al. 2013). First, impairment in the formation of solid and stable granulomas prevents the containment of the infection, and second, it prevents the development of clinically diagnosable symptoms of TB. One study found the death rate of smokers with TB to be nine times higher than that of nonsmokers with TB. Of those smokers who died the majority did not report symptoms associated with TB prior to diagnosis as opposed to the nonsmokers (Wen et al. 2010). Another potential factor that could increase TB mortality from CS would be the decreased effectiveness of TB treatment in active smokers (Chiang et al. 2012).

Cigarette Smoking and TB Recurrence

To date, the evidence implicating CS with increased rates of TB recurrence is suggestive of a causal relationship, but additional research is still required. One of the more comprehensive studies found that CS only slightly increased the risk of TB recurrence in men (hazard ratio [HR] = 1.3; 95% CI, 1.2–1.4) with a similar, although even slighter, risk for women (HR = 1.2; 95% CI, 0.8–1.6) (Jee et al. 2009). Other studies have been conducted indicating a correlation between the two with an OR as high as 3.1 (OR = 3.1; 95% CI, 1.6–6.0) (Thomas et al. 2005; d'Arc Lyra Batista et al. 2008; Leung et al. 2004).

Cigarette Smoking and *M. tb* Infection

The Surgeon General Report found the evidence implicating CS and increased risks for *M. tb* infection is inconclusive. To date, majority of research has been conducted via cross-sectional studies that do not allow for the analysis of the sequence of causation or the relationship between CS and TB (Surgeon General Report 2014). Additionally, we do not have supporting evidence indicating a dose-response relationship between vulnerability to *M. tb* infection and CS. However, previous studies have strongly implicated CS as a causative factor in increased susceptibility to an initial *M. tb* infection, and the need for additional research has been legitimized. With the previous limitations in mind, the available studies have shown that smokers are a greater risk for susceptibility to *M. tb* infection than nonsmokers (RR = 1.2–2.7) (Surgeon General Report 2014). A study in South Africa found that when exposed to *M. tb* infection and CS in tandem the increased risk is staggering.

Children who lived in a household with an active TB case and who were also exposed to CS showed a dramatic increase in susceptibility to infection (OR = 4.60; 95% CI, 1.29–16.45) (den Boon et al. 2007). This strongly implicates the importance of the immune system's function in protecting the host from initial infection and also implicates the veracity of research purporting the immune system-compromising effects of the smoke-induced suppression of ciliary epithelial cell function (Altet et al. 1996). The results are considered inconclusive due to the limited number of investigations and also the need for adjustment to more variables (SES and demographic factors) and also to the differentiation between reactivation of latent TB and secondary exogenous *M. tb* infection.

Although additional research analyzing the relationship that CS has on the TB life cycle and mechanism of infection is required, the supporting literature is sufficient to indict CS as a risk factor for both those currently diagnosed with TB and those at risk of exposure. Immediate action should be taken to implement smoking cessation into the treatment plan of infected and recovering individuals and more broadly for increased education in at risk demographics of the susceptibility-inducing effects of smoking. Additionally, the need is dire for research into the variety of mechanisms of the immunocompromising effects of CS, thereby allowing for advances in prevention and treatment options. Lastly, additional long-term studies are necessary to explore the correlation between TB pathology and CS.

Oxidative Stress

To better understand the linkage of CS's effect on the ability of the immune system to combat *M. tb* infection, we must first establish the groundwork for one of the most significant mechanisms it is purported to use for immunocompromisation, namely, oxidative stress. Oxidative stress has been implicated in the pathogenesis of hypertension (Rodrigo et al. 2011), diabetes type 2 (Henriksen et al. 2011), schizophrenia (Grabnar et al. 2011), carcinogenesis (Klaunig et al. 2009), heart failure (Tsutsui et al. 2011), and neurodegeneration (Kim et al. 2015). That is not to say that oxidative stress is a single variable problem as the maintenance of balance in the host's redox system is essential to health, and the excess production of antioxidants is linked to pathologies of its own (Sies et al. 2017). For our purposes, however, we will primarily focus our attention on the increased OS caused by CS and the mechanisms by which CS compromises the immune system to *M. tb*. The topics briefly touched on below are not comprehensive as OS has systemic effects on both the innate and adaptive immune systems, which we will briefly touch on later, but this section is intended to be a superficial examination of primary mechanisms.

Antioxidants

One of the best ways to study the mechanisms by which oxidative stress taxes the immune system is by reversing the problem and studying the immune-bolstering effects of antioxidants. You will remember from earlier in this book that significant research has been done linking the systemic effects of oxidative stress and the increased susceptibility to TB infection (Morris et al. 2013). As a result of this causal relationship, research has been conducted to explore the potential immune-bolstering effects of antioxidants. Two of the primary roles of antioxidants that have been discovered are their roles in redox balance and their antimicrobial properties (Sies et al. 2017).

One of the important roles that antioxidants play in the maintenance of a healthy immune system is by acting as a buffer for the natural killer molecules produced by the immune system. The "killer molecules" are primarily radical oxygen species (ROS) and reactive nitrogen intermediates (RNI) (Islamoglu et al. 2018). These molecules are produced by macrophages during phagocytosis and use their reactivity to neutralize any internalized pathogens. However, these cells are so reactive that they can be detrimental to the host's health as well if a corresponding amount of antioxidants—such as glutathione (GSH)—are not produced. Without antioxidants the collateral damage caused by the immune system's response to infection could expose the host to increased susceptibility to additional infections. Antioxidants buffering the redox equation and maintaining balance are also essential because of the redox signaling pathway. The proper functioning of which is essential to immune system function and which if artificially altered outside the physiological standard limits could have systemic effects on the immune system. This could be caused by both excess of oxidants and antioxidants (Niki 2016).

Antioxidants are also important antimicrobials. For our purposes we will examine the many roles of GSH as an example since it is one of the most studied antioxidants. It has been demonstrated to have direct antimycobacterial properties (Zhang and Duan 2009; Schairer et al. 2013). Furthermore, GSH can act as a substrate for NO to form S-nitrosoglutathione (GSNO) which serves as a NO donor; release of NO from GSNO complex can result in the killing of the pathogen. Also, GSH has been shown to have antimycobacterial effects on its own without NO. Although the mechanism is not well-understood, it has been suggested that the primary mechanism of GSH killing mycobacteria could be the shift in the redox balance. The presence of GSH in high concentrations plus the cell's natural concentration of an alternative thiol (mycothiol) that acts as an antioxidant might cause the delicate balance to shift (Venketaraman et al. 2006). Due to these antibiotic-like functions, some researchers have compared GSH to the precursor of the Penicillin and its potential conversion to a derivative of a penicillin-like molecule known as glutacillin (Morris et al. 2013). Due to the structural similarities and functional comparisons, GSH has also been shown to be necessary in the effective functioning of the natural killer cells (NK) (Morris et al. 2013). The killing of intracellular pathogens by NK cells has been shown to be dependent on GSH concentrations.

These examples are but a sample of the host of roles that antioxidants play in the regulation of a healthy immune system and they establish an interesting field of inquiry into a mechanism of CS effect on the immune system. Namely, does CS increase oxidative stress, overwhelm the natural antioxidants of the host's immune system, and deplete the reservoir of GSH?

Smoking and Oxidative Stress

Cigarette smoke is a cocktail of more than 4700 ingredients that include among its constituent chemicals from ammonia, to nitrogen oxides, to hydrogen cyanide, to trace metals (Kamceva et al. 2016). For our purposes we will be most concerned with those constituents which are also ROS. Due to these ROS both cellular reactive oxygen species (cROS) and mitochondrial reactive oxygen species (mtROS) have been shown to increase after exposure to cigarette smoke extract (CSE) (Valdivieso et al. 2018). Increased ROS is especially problematic for the immune system when found in the mitochondria. This is because mtROS has been shown to damage mtDNA and impair mitochondrial proteins (Valdivieso et al. 2018; Liang and Godley 2003; Darley-Usmar and Kramer 2015). The role of mitochondria in the oxidative phosphorylation system (OXPHOS) indicates that damage caused by mtROS could have cascading effects on the host's ability to control ROS production which might lead to additional oxidative stress, thus initiating a cycle of oxidative damage.

Some of the mechanisms by which CS has been linked to increased OS would include the following. CS's nitric oxide reacts with alkenes in the smoke to form carbon-centered radicals (Yao and Keshavan 2011). Radical chemical agents found in smoke are known as semiquinones. Semiquinone is a general term for a radical which is formed via the loss of a hydrogen atom and corresponding electron and which will increase the concentration of hydrogen peroxide. Also, CS has been studied for its relationship to albumin, bilirubin, and thioredoxin which are three important proteins in the redox system. Albumin and bilirubin are important free radical-scavenging proteins, and thioredoxin is a redox-regulating protein that also has antioxidant activity (Nakamura 2005; Yao and Keshavan 2011). Of these three only bilirubin concentration has been correlated with CS (Yao et al. 2000), and bilirubin by itself only accounts for <5% of the overall contribution of plasma total antioxidant status (TAS). Therefore, CS is not thought to actively increase OS by affecting the concentration of these three proteins.

Nicotine deserves special consideration as there appears to be disagreement in the literature over its effect on the redox balance. Nicotine has been shown to substantially increase ROS (Barr et al. 2007). Mesencephalic cells incubated with concentrations of nicotine as small as 0.1 μM increased ROS by approximately 35% and concentrations of 1 and 10 μM increased ROS by 54% and 80%, respectively (Barr et al. 2007). Nicotine has also been shown to cause oxidative tissue damage in rats (Husain et al. 2001) and significantly deplete the reserves of GSH in the liver and testes of male rats. Also, nicotine is purported to increase free radical concentrations by activating neutrophils. Conversely, nicotine has also been investigated for antioxidant properties. Particularly, in its relation to purported protective effects against Alzheimer's and Parkinson's disease (Linert et al. 1999; Ferger et al. 1998; Yao et al. 2011). These conflicting findings in addition to additional investigation have led some researchers to believe that cigarette smoke's cacophony of ingredients may counteract each other and ultimately have little effect on the antioxidant defense system (AODS) of the host (Yao et al. 2011).

Research has also been done to study whether this OS caused by CS is reversible. Two different compounds have been used including both GSH and N-acetyl Cysteine (NAC)—the rate-limiting reactant in the formation of GSH. The observed results were the modulation of biochemical marker enzyme LDH, the decrease of lipid peroxidation, and a generalized increase in the host's antioxidant reserves (Dey and Roy 2010).

Oxidative Stress and Tuberculosis

The potential for OS to compromise the immune system has been well-documented. As it relates to the specific mechanisms by which it affects the host's ability to combat *M. tb* infection, we will speak more specifically in the following sections. Regarding TB mortality, it has also been well-documented that the immune system's defense against *M. tb* infection causes an increase in the oxidative stress on the host (Torun et al. 2014). Likely, this is due to the increased production of ROS by the immune system in a targeted attempt to eliminate the invading pathogen (Voskuil et al. 2011). Although necessary, this increase in ROS in response to *M. tb* infection could be problematic when coupled with the purported tax on the redox balance that CS causes. A resulting shift in the redox balance could ensue causing a fallout effect, increasing necrosis of localized tissue and potentially damaging the delicate redox signaling mechanism thereby initiating systemic effects on the control of the infection (Islamoglu et al. 2018; Murphy et al. 2017; Brooker 2011). This is a mechanistic explanation for the increase of TB mortality that CS has.

Cigarette Smoking and the Immune System's Defense Against Tuberculosis

To summarize our understanding of the immunocompromising effects of CS—especially as it relates to increased susceptibility to *M. tb* infection—we will review the specific mechanisms by which CS has been shown to compromise the innate and adaptive immune systems. We can do this both by appreciating those specific mechanisms of protection that CS has been shown to impede and also by drawing some generalized conclusions from those effects of oxidative stress that we have already shown CS to have.

Innate Immune System

The innate immune system can be thought of as the first line of defense against invasion. It prevents infection first by a system of physical barriers like skin, saliva, mucus, etc. and secondarily by a chemical barrier of antimicrobial substances, e.g., antimicrobial proteins and peptides (Owen et al. 2013). If a pathogen circumnavigates these first two, it is then met with the innate system's last resort which is a barrage of instantaneous cellular responses that attempt to overwhelm the invasion via a complex system of macrophages, fluid, antimicrobials, and necessary nutrients of the defensive cohort. Colloquially, this response is referred to as inflammation.

Cigarette smoke has been implicated in the disruption of the first two protective mechanisms. For example, in the disruption of ciliary function necessary to the movement and excretion of mucus, thus exposing the host to an increased risk to infection and a path of less resistance to the organism's end goal, the alveoli (Arcavi and Benowitz 2004). Also, CS has been implicated in pathologies that directly affect the epithelial cells protecting the interior of the lung's surfaces, which are crucial in the protection from various antigens (U.S. Department of Health 2010). Two examples of pathologies for which cigarette smoking is a well-documented primary risk factor would be chronic obstructive pulmonary disease (COPD) (Laniado-Laborín 2009) and idiopathic pulmonary fibrosis (IPF) (Baumgartner et al. 1997; Chad et al. 2012; Connell and Venketaraman 2009) which impair lung health, alter tissue, and could very plausibly impair this first line of defense.

Although these effects on the first two barriers to infection are important, it is in the realm of the third line—that of the cellular responses—that we see the most potential for a mechanistic explanation of cigarette smoke's detrimental effects on the workings of the innate immune system. Nicotine present in cigarette smoke has been shown to impede the ability of macrophages to combat TB (Bai et al. 2017). Also, cigarette smoke has been shown to impede the response of alveolar macrophages (Gaschler et al. 2008). Cigarette smoke extract has been observed to increase production of cytokines IL-6 and IL-8 which are primarily responsible for increased inflammation and chemotaxis (Valdivieso et al. 2018). This effect has been demonstrated to be reversible by administration of NAC, which indicates that the spike in cytokine production is controlled by ROS signaling (Cazzola et al. 2017; Comer et al. 2014; Ko et al. 2015; Wu et al. 2017; Zhou et al. 2016). Another mechanism of immunocompromisation due to cigarette smoking is the decreased functioning ability of lysosomes because of the intracellular accumulation of cigarette smoke debris (Meijer and Aerts 2016; Vergne et al. 2004; Lee et al. 2012; Hodge et al. 2003; Kirkham et al. 2004). Lysosomes are a crucial player in the innate system's containment of TB as they bind to the phagosomes after the bacilli have been phagocytized and release a chemical concoction that destroys the pathogen. This detrimental effect of CS on the phagocytic process mimics the natural evasion mechanism of *M. tb* which is to prevent phagosome maturation lysosome binding. As briefly mentioned earlier CS has also been implicated in delayed diagnosis of TB and in the impaired formation of solid and stable granulomas.

Adaptive Immune System

After the initial infection is phagocytized, the bacilli are very resilient to destruction and will continue to proliferate intracellularly. If the innate system has failed to control the infection, the host will, as a second choice to annihilation of the intracellular pathogen, produce cytokines from CD4$^+$ T cells (T$_H$1 subset). This is where the adaptive immune system's role begins.

The cytokines produced will facilitate the more effective suppression—and sometimes destruction—of the intracellular pathogens. A particularly important cytokine would be IFN-γ, which has been demonstrated to be especially important in the suppression of *M. tb* infection (Owen et al. 2013). An insightful study demonstrated that mice without the ability to produce IFN-γ were highly susceptible to even an attenuated strain of mycobacteria, whereas the wild type mice survived. Significantly, CS has been shown to impede this response mechanism and decrease cytokine production, including that of IFN-γ (Phaybouth et al. 2006; Vassallo et al. 2005; Shaler et al. 2013; Shang et al. 2011; Feng et al. 2011). CS has also been implicated in the suppression of type I by the downregulation of Th1 cytokines and the preferential production of Th2 cytokines thereby exposing the host to increased susceptibility of certain bacterial and viral pathogens usually contained via the production of Th1 cytokines (Shaler et al. 2013; Phaybouth et al. 2006; Vassallo et al. 2005; Shang et al. 2011). *M. tb* is one such pathogen which ostensibly utilizes this vulnerability thus explaining the increased mortality of cigarette smokers (Fig. 1).

The mechanisms by which CS has been demonstrated to impair the adaptive immune system's ability to contain *M. tb* are no less comprehensive than those

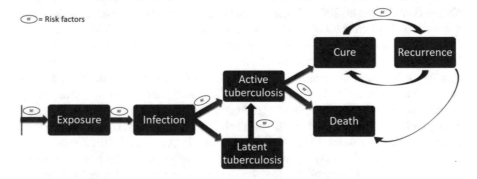

Fig. 1 CS and increased susceptibility to TB

demonstrated for the innate. Besides decreasing cytokine production, another potential mechanism by which CS impairs the adaptive immune system is via the GSH-depleting effects that the oxidative stress associated with cigarette smoke (as discussed previously) can have. Low GSH levels have been implicated in decreased levels of Th1 cytokines leading to successful growth and replication of *M. tb* (Guerra et al. 2011). And yet another study demonstrated that the aggravation of continuous cigarette smoke will mitigate the localized recruitment of CD4 + IFN-γ + T cells which is obviously essential to the first response of the immune system.

Summary

Besides those effects which conveniently fall within the separate spheres of innate and adaptive immunity, there are also systemic effects which bridge the gap between these two systems. The decreased production of TNF, IL-12, and RANTES, as well as the accumulation of APCs due to CS would be some such examples (Shaler et al. 2013).

References

Altet, M. N., Alcaide, J., Plans, P., Taberner, J. L., Salto, E., Folguera, L. I., & Salleras, L. (1996). Passive smoking and risk of pulmonary tuberculosis in children immediately following infection. A case-control study. *Tubercle and Lung Disease, 77*(6), 537–544.

Arcavi, L., & Benowitz, N. L. (2004). Cigarette smoking and infection. *Archives of Internal Medicine, 164*(20), 2206.

Bai, X., et al. (2017). Nicotine impairs macrophage control of Mycobacterium tuberculosis. *Advances in Pediatrics*. Available at: https://www.ncbi.nlm.nih.gov/pubmed/28398760. Accessed 15 May 2018.

Barr, J., et al. (2007). Nicotine induces oxidative stress and activates nuclear transcription factor kappa B in rat mesencephalic cells. *Advances in Pediatrics*. Available at: https://www.ncbi.nlm.nih.gov/pmc/articles/PMC2758082/. Accessed 14 May 2018.

Baumgartner, K. B., et al. (1997). Cigarette smoking: A risk factor for idiopathic pulmonary fibrosis. *Advances in Pediatrics*. Available at: https://www.ncbi.nlm.nih.gov/pubmed/9001319. Accessed 15 May 2018.

Bronner Murrison, L., Martinson, N., Moloney, R., Msandiwa, R., Mashabela, M., Samet, J., & Golub, J. (2016). Tobacco smoking and tuberculosis among men living with HIV in Johannesburg, South Africa: A case-control study. *PLoS One, 11*(11), e0167133.

Brooker, R. J. (2011). *Genetics: Analysis and principles*. New York, NY: McGraw-Hill Science.

Cazzola, M., et al. (2017). Pharmacological investigation on the anti-oxidant and anti-inflammatory activity of N-acetylcysteine in an ex vivo model of COPD exacerbation. *Respiratory Research, 18*(1), 26.

Chad, K., Murray, A., & Nestor, N. (2012). Smoking and idiopathic pulmonary fibrosis. *International Scholarly Research Notices*. Available at: https://www.hindawi.com/journals/pm/2012/808260/. Accessed 15 May 2018.

Chiang, Y., Lin, Y., Lee, J., Lee, C., & Chen, H. (2012). Tobacco consumption is a reversible risk factor associated with reduced successful treatment outcomes of anti-tuberculosis therapy. *International Journal of Infectious Diseases, 16*(2), e130–e135.

Comer, D. M., Elborn, J. S., & Ennis, M. (2014). Inflammatory and cytotoxic effects of acrolein, nicotine, acetylaldehyde and cigarette smoke extract on human nasal epithelial cells. *BMC Pulmonary Medicine, 14*(1), 32.

Connell, N., & Venketaraman, V. (2009). Control of Mycobacterium tuberculosis infection by glutathione. *Recent Patents on Anti-Infective Drug Discovery, 4*(3), 214–226.

d'Arc Lyra Batista, J., de Fátima Pessoa Militão de Albuquerque, M., de Alencar Ximenes, R. A., & Rodrigues, L. C. (2008). Smoking increases the risk of relapse after successful tuberculosis treatment. *International Journal of Epidemiology, 37*(4), 841–851.

Darley-Usmar, V., & Kramer, P. (2015). The emerging theme of redox bioenergetics in health and disease. *Biomedical Journal, 38*(4), 294.

den Boon, S., Verver, S., Marais, B. J., Enarson, D. A., Lombard, C. J., Bateman, E. D., Irusen, E., Jithoo, A., Gie, R. P., Borgdorff, M. W., et al. (2007). Association between passive smoking and infection with Mycobacterium tuberculosis in children. *Pediatrics, 119*(4), 734–739.

Dey, S. K., & Roy, S. (2010). Role of reduced glutathione in the amelioration of nicotine-induced oxidative stress. *Advances in Pediatrics*. Available at: https://www.ncbi.nlm.nih.gov/pubmed/20221824. Accessed 14 May 2018.

Feng, Y., et al. (2011). Exposure to cigarette smoke inhibits the pulmonary T-cell response to influenza virus and Mycobacterium tuberculosis. *Advances in Pediatrics*. Available at: https://www.ncbi.nlm.nih.gov/pmc/articles/PMC3019896/. Accessed 15 May 2018.

Ferger, B., et al. (1998). Effects of nicotine on hydroxyl free radical formation in vitro and on MPTP-induced neurotoxicity in vivo. *Advances in Pediatrics*. Available at: https://www.ncbi.nlm.nih.gov/pubmed/9774223/. Accessed 14 May 2018.

Gajalakshmi, V., Peto, R., Kanaka, T. S., & Jha, P. (2003). Smoking and mortality from tuberculosis and other diseases in India: Retrospective study of 43000 adult male deaths and 35000 controls. *Lancet, 362*(9383), 507–515.

Gaschler, G. J., et al. (2008). Cigarette smoke exposure attenuates cytokine production by mouse alveolar macrophages. *Advances in Pediatrics*. Available at: https://www.ncbi.nlm.nih.gov/pubmed/17872497. Accessed 15 May 2018.

Grabnar, I., Vovk, T., Kores Plesnicar, B., & Boskovic, M. (2011). Oxidative stress in schizophrenia. *Current Neuropharmacology, 9*(2), 301–312.

Guerra, C., et al. (2011). Glutathione and adaptive immune responses against Mycobacterium tuberculosis infection in healthy and HIV infected individuals. *Advances in Pediatrics*. Available at: https://www.ncbi.nlm.nih.gov/pubmed/22164280. Accessed 15 May 2018.

Henriksen, E., Diamond-Stanic, M., & Marchionne, E. (2011). Oxidative stress and the etiology of insulin resistance and type 2 diabetes. *Free Radical Biology and Medicine, 51*(5), 993–999.

Hodge, S., et al. (2003). Alveolar macrophages from subjects with chronic obstructive pulmonary disease are deficient in their ability to phagocytose apoptotic airway epithelial cells. *Advances in Pediatrics*. Available at: https://www.ncbi.nlm.nih.gov/pubmed/12848850/. Accessed 15 May 2018.

Husain, K., et al. (2001). Chronic ethanol and nicotine interaction on rat tissue antioxidant defense system. *Advances in Pediatrics*. Available at: https://www.ncbi.nlm.nih.gov/pubmed/11747978. Accessed 14 May 2018.

Islamoglu, H., et al. (2018). Effects of ReadiSorb L-GSH in altering granulomatous responses against Mycobacterium tuberculosis infection. *Journal of Clinical Medicine, 7*(3), 40.

Jee, S. H., Golub, J. E., Jo, J., Park, I. S., Ohrr, H., & Samet, J. M. (2009). Smoking and risk of tuberculosis incidence, mortality, and recurrence in South Korean men and women. *American Journal of Epidemiology, 170*(12), 1478–1485.

Jha, P., Jacob, B., Gajalakshmi, V., Gupta, P. C., Dhingra, N., Kumar, R., Sinha, D. N., Dikshit, R. P., Parida, D. K., Kamadod, R., et al. (2008). A nationally representative case-control study of smoking and death in India. *New England Journal of Medicine, 358*(11), 1137–1147.

Kamceva, G., et al. (2016). Cigarette smoking and oxidative stress in patients with coronary artery disease. *Advances in Pediatrics*. Available at: https://www.ncbi.nlm.nih.gov/pmc/articles/PMC5175512/#ref2. Accessed 14 May 2018.

Kim, G. H., et al. (2015). The role of oxidative stress in neurodegenerative diseases. *Advances in Pediatrics*. Available at: https://www.ncbi.nlm.nih.gov/pmc/articles/PMC4688332/. Accessed 14 May 2018.

Kirkham, P. A., et al. (2004). Macrophage phagocytosis of apoptotic neutrophils is compromised by matrix proteins modified by cigarette smoke and lipid peroxidation products. *Advances in Pediatrics*. Available at: https://www.ncbi.nlm.nih.gov/pubmed/15110749/. Accessed 15 May 2018.

Klaunig, J. E., Kamendulis, L. M., & Hocevar, B. A. (2009). Oxidative stress and oxidative damage in carcinogenesis. *Toxicologic Pathology, 38*(1), 96–109.

Ko, H.-K., et al. (2015). Regulation of cigarette smoke induction of IL-8 in macrophages by AMP-activated protein kinase signaling. *Journal of Cellular Physiology, 230*(8), 1781–1793.

Kuemmerer, J. M., & Comstock, G. W. (1967). Sociologic concomitants of tuberculin sensitivity. *American Review of Respiratory Disease, 96*(5), 885–892.

Lam, T. H., Ho, S. Y., Hedley, A. J., Mak, K. H., & Peto, R. (2001). Mortality and smoking in Hong Kong: Case-control study of all adult deaths in 1998. *British Medical Journal, 323*(7309), 361.

Laniado-Laborín, R. (2009). Smoking and chronic obstructive pulmonary disease (COPD). Parallel epidemics of the 21st century. *Advances in Pediatrics*. Available at: https://www.ncbi.nlm.nih.gov/pmc/articles/PMC2672326/. Accessed 15 May 2018.

Lee, J., Taneja, V., & Vassallo, R. (2012). Cigarette smoking and inflammation cellular and molecular mechanisms. *Advances in Pediatrics*. Available at: https://www.ncbi.nlm.nih.gov/pmc/articles/PMC3261116/. Accessed 15 May 2018.

Leung, C. C., Li, T., Lam, T. H., Yew, W. W., Law, W. S., Tam, C. M., Chan, W. M., Chan, C. K., Ho, K. S., & Chang, K. C. (2004). Smoking and tuberculosis among the elderly in Hong Kong. *American Journal of Respiratory and Critical Care Medicine, 170*(9), 1027–1033.

Liang, F.-Q., & Godley, B. F. (2003). Oxidative stress-induced mitochondrial DNA damage in human retinal pigment epithelial cells: A possible mechanism for RPE aging and age-related macular degeneration. *Experimental Eye Research, 76*(4), 397–403.

Lin, H. H., Ezzati, M., Chang, H. Y., & Murray, M. (2009). Association between tobacco smoking and active tuberculosis in Taiwan: Prospective cohort study. *American Journal of Respiratory and Critical Care Medicine, 180*(5), 475–480.

Linert, W., et al. (1999). In vitro and in vivo studies investigating possible antioxidant actions of nicotine: Relevance to Parkinson's and Alzheimer's diseases. *Advances in Pediatrics*. Available at: https://www.ncbi.nlm.nih.gov/pubmed/10381559/. Accessed 14 May 2018.

Liu, B. Q., Peto, R., Chen, Z. M., Boreham, J., Wu, Y. P., Li, J. Y., Campbell, T. C., & Chen, J. S. (1998). Emerging tobacco hazards in China: 1. Retrospective proportional mortality study of one million deaths. *British Medical Journal, 317*(7170), 1411–1422.

Lönnroth, K., Williams, B. G., Cegielski, P., & Dye, C. (2010). A consistent log-linear relationship between tuberculosis incidence and body mass index. *Int J Epidemiol, 39*(1), 149–155.

Lönnroth, K., et al. (2018). Tuberculosis control and elimination 2010–50: Cure, care, and social development. *Lancet*. Available at: https://www.ncbi.nlm.nih.gov/pubmed/20488524. Accessed 10 May 2018.

Meijer, A. Â. H., & Aerts, J. Â. M. (2016). Linking smokers' susceptibility to tuberculosis with lysosomal storage disorders. *Developmental Cell, 37*(2), 112–113.

Morris, D., et al. (2013). Glutathione and infection. *Biochimica et Biophysica Acta (BBA) - General Subjects, 1830*(5), 3329–3349.

Murphy, K. M., et al. (2017). *Janeway's immunobiology*. New York, NY: Garland Science, Taylor & Francis Group.

Nakamura, H. (2005). Thioredoxin and its related molecules: Update 2005. *Advances in Pediatrics*. Available at: https://www.ncbi.nlm.nih.gov/pubmed/15890030/. Accessed 14 May 2018.

Niki, E. (2016). Oxidative stress and antioxidants: Distress or eustress? *Archives of Biochemistry and Biophysics, 595,* 19–24.

Owen, J., Punt, J., Stranford, S., & Jones, P. (2013). *Kuby immunology.* New York, NY: W.H. Freeman.

Phaybouth, V., et al. (2006). Cigarette smoke suppresses Th1 cytokine production and increases RSV expression in a neonatal model. *Advances in Pediatrics.* Available at: https://www.ncbi. nlm.nih.gov/pubmed/16126789/. Accessed 15 May 2018.

Prasad, R., Garg, R., Singhal, S., Dawar, R., & Agarwal, G. G. (2009). A case control study of tobacco smoking and tuberculosis in India. *Annals of Thoracic Medicine, 4*(4), 208–210.

Rodrigo, R., González, J., & Paoletto, F. (2011). The role of oxidative stress in the pathophysiology of hypertension. *Hypertension Research, 34*(4), 431–440.

Samet, J. M. (2018). Tobacco smoking: the leading cause of preventable disease worldwide. *Thoracic Surgery Clinics.* Available at: https://www.ncbi.nlm.nih.gov/pubmed/23566962. Accessed 10 May 2018.

Schairer, D. O., et al. (2013). Evaluation of the antibiotic properties of glutathione. *Advances in Pediatrics.* Available at: https://www.ncbi.nlm.nih.gov/pubmed/24196336. Accessed 14 May 2018.

Shaler, C. R., et al. (2013). Continuous and discontinuous cigarette smoke exposure differentially affects protective Th1 immunity against pulmonary tuberculosis. *Advances in Pediatrics.* Available at: https://www.ncbi.nlm.nih.gov/pmc/articles/PMC3602464/. Accessed 15 May 2018.

Shang, S., et al. (2011). Cigarette smoke increases susceptibility to tuberculosis-evidence from in vivo and in vitro models. *The Journal of Infectious Diseases.* Available at: https://academic. oup.com/jid/article/203/9/1240/2192103. Accessed 15 May 2018.

Sies, H., Berndt, C., & Jones, D. P. (2017). Oxidative stress. *Annual Review of Biochemistry, 86*(1), 715–748.

Sitas, F., Urban, M., Bradshaw, D., Kielkowski, D., Bah, S., & Peto, R. (2004). Tobacco attributable deaths in South Africa. *Tobacco Control, 13*(4), 396–399.

Slama, K., et al. (2018). Tobacco and tuberculosis: a qualitative systematic review and meta-analysis. *International Journal of Tuberculosis and Lung Disease.* Available at: https://www. ncbi.nlm.nih.gov/pubmed/17945060. Accessed 10 May 2018.

Smith, G. S., et al. (2018). Cigarette smoking and pulmonary tuberculosis in northern California. *Journal of Epidemiology and Community Health.* Available at: https://www.ncbi.nlm.nih.gov/ pubmed/25605864. Accessed 13 May 2018.

Smoking and Tobacco Use. (2018). *CDC – fact sheet – fast facts – smoking & tobacco use.* Available at: https://www.cdc.gov/tobacco/data_statistics/fact_sheets

Thomas, A., Gopi, P. G., Santha, T., Chandrasekaran, V., Subramani, R., Selvakumar, N., Eusuff, S. I., Sadacharam, K., & Narayanan, P. R. (2005). Predictors of relapse among pulmonary tuberculosis patients treated in a DOTS programme in South India. *The International Journal of Tuberculosis and Lung Disease, 9*(5), 556–561.

Torun, E., et al. (2014). Serum paraoxonase 1 activity and oxidative stress in pediatric patients with pulmonary tuberculosis. *Advances in Pediatrics.* Available at: https://www.ncbi.nlm.nih.gov/ pmc/articles/PMC5586969/. Accessed 14 May 2018.

Tsutsui, H., Kinugawa, S., & Matsushima, S. (2011). Oxidative stress and heart failure. *Advances in Pediatrics.* Available at: https://www.ncbi.nlm.nih.gov/pubmed/21949114. Accessed 14 May 2018.

U.S. Department of Health and Human Services. (2014). *The health consequences of smoking: 50 years of progress. A report of the Surgeon General.* Atlanta, GA: U.S. Department of Health and Human Services, Centers for Disease Control and Prevention, National Center for Chronic Disease Prevention and Health Promotion, Office on Smoking and Health. Printed with corrections, January 2014.

U.S. Department of Health and Human Services, Centers for Disease Control and Prevention, National Center for and Health Promotion. (2010). *How tobacco smoke causes disease:*

The biology and behavioral basis for smoking-attributable disease: A report of the Surgeon General. Rockville, MD: U.S. Department of Health and Human Services, Public Health Service, Office of the Surgeon General.

Valdivieso, Ã. G., et al. (2018). N-acetyl cysteine reverts the proinflammatory state induced by cigarette smoke extract in lung Calu-3 cells. *Redox Biology, 16*, 294–302.

Vassallo, R., et al. (2005). Cigarette smoke extract suppresses human dendritic cell function leading to preferential induction of Th-2 priming. *Advances in Pediatrics*. Available at: https://www.ncbi.nlm.nih.gov/pubmed/16081845/. Accessed 15 May 2018.

Venketaraman, V., et al. (2006). Glutathione and growth inhibition of Mycobacterium tuberculosis in healthy and HIV infected subjects. *AIDS Research and Therapy, 3*, 5. Available at: https://aidsrestherapy.biomedcentral.com/articles/10.1186/1742-6405-3-5#Sec14. Accessed 14 May 2018.

Vergne, I., et al. (2004). Cell biology of mycobacterium tuberculosis phagosome. *Advances in Pediatrics*. Available at: https://www.ncbi.nlm.nih.gov/pubmed/15473845. Accessed 15 May 2018.

Voskuil, M. I., et al. (2011). The response of mycobacterium tuberculosis to reactive oxygen and nitrogen species. *Advances in Pediatrics*. Available at: https://www.ncbi.nlm.nih.gov/pubmed/21734908. Accessed 14 May 2018.

Webb, G. B. (1918). The effect of the inhalation of cigarette smoke on the lungs. A clinical study. *American Review of Tuberculosis, 1*, 25–27.

Wen, C., Chan, T., Chan, H., Tsai, M., Cheng, T., & Tsai, S. (2010). The reduction of tuberculosis risks by smoking cessation. *BMC Infectious Diseases, 10*(1), 156.

WHO report on the global tobacco epidemic (2017). 1–244.

World Health Organization. (2018a). *Global tuberculosis report*. Available at: http://www.who.int/tb/publications/global_report/en/. Accessed 13 May 2018.

World Health Organization Framework Convention on Tobacco Control. (2010). *Analysis of the available technology for unique markings in view of the global track and trace regime proposed in the negotiating text for a protocol to eliminate illicit trade in tobacco products*. Available at: http://apps.who.int/gb/fctc/PDF/it4/FCTC_COP_INB_ IT4_ID1-en.pdf. Accessed 10 May 2018.

Wu, Y. P., et al. (2017). Activating transcription factor 3 represses cigarette smoke-induced IL6 and IL8 expression via suppressing NF-κB activation. *Advances in Pediatrics*. Available at: https://www.ncbi.nlm.nih.gov/pubmed/28185985. Accessed 15 May 2018.

Yao, J. K., & Keshavan, M. S. (2011). Antioxidants, redox signaling, and pathophysiology in schizophrenia: An integrative view. *Advances in Pediatrics*. Available at: https://www.ncbi.nlm.nih.gov/pmc/articles/PMC3159108/. Accessed 14 May 2018.

Yao, S., Huang, W. H., van den Hof, S., Yang, S. M., Wang, X. L., Chen, W., Fang, X. H., & Pan, H. F. (2011). Treatment adherence among sputum smear-positive pulmonary tuberculosis patients in mountainous areas in China. *BMC Health Serv Res, 11*, 341.

Yao, J. K., Reddy, R., & van Kammen, D. P. (2000). Abnormal age-related changes of plasma antioxidant proteins in schizophrenia. *Advances in Pediatrics*. Available at: https://www.ncbi.nlm.nih.gov/pubmed/11166086. Accessed 14 May 2018.

Yu, G. P., Hsieh, C. C., & Peng, J. (1988). Risk factors associated with the prevalence of pulmonary tuberculosis among sanitary workers in Shanghai. *Tubercle, 69*(2), 105–112.

Zhang, Y., & Duan, K. (2009). Glutathione exhibits antibacterial activity and increases tetracycline efficacy against Pseudomonas aeruginosa. *Advances in Pediatrics*. Available at: https://www.ncbi.nlm.nih.gov/pubmed/19557326. Accessed 14 May 2018.

Zhou, G., et al. (2016). Chemical constituents of tobacco smoke induce the production of interleukin-8 in human bronchial epithelium, 16HBE cells. *Tobacco Induced Diseases, 14*(1), 24.

Coinfection with *Mycobacterium tuberculosis* and HIV

Luke Elizabeth Hanna

Epidemiology of TB and HIV

Dual infection with *Mycobacterium tuberculosis* (MTB) and Human Immunodeficiency Virus (HIV) has become an alarming problem that poses major challenges to health care, particularly in developing countries. The World Health Organization (WHO) estimated 10.4 million new cases of active TB globally in 2016, of which 10% was among people living with HIV. Approximately 374,000 deaths were reported among those with TB and HIV coinfection in the same year (WHO 2017).

There is a complex relationship between infection with TB and HIV that results in a synergistic increase in their prevalence, morbidity, and mortality. Infection with HIV is the most powerful risk factor for acquisition of MTB infection and disease progression. The risk of developing TB is estimated to be 16–27 times greater in people living with HIV than among those without HIV infection (WHO 2018). While the estimated lifetime risk of progression from latent to active TB in HIV negative people is about 5–10%, for HIV infected individuals this becomes the annual risk (WHO 2008). Even so, TB is the leading cause of death among HIV-infected individuals, accounting for about 26% of AIDS-related deaths (WHO 2009a). Due to the risks associated with coinfection, the Centres for Disease Control (CDC) recommends that all persons living with HIV be tested for TB and that those with latent TB infection be initiated on anti-TB treatment (WHO 2018).

L. E. Hanna (✉)
National Institute for Research in Tuberculosis, Chennai, India
e-mail: hanna@nirt.res.in

© Springer Nature Switzerland AG 2018
V. Venketaraman (ed.), *Understanding the Host Immune Response Against Mycobacterium tuberculosis Infection*, https://doi.org/10.1007/978-3-319-97367-8_7

Epidemiology of Multidrug-Resistant (MDR) TB and Extensively Drug-Resistant (XDR) TB Among HIV-Infected Persons

There is very limited data on the global epidemiology of drug-resistant TB in HIV-infected persons. Although earlier studies reported no association between MDR-TB and HIV infection (Kenyon et al. 1999; Chum et al. 1996; Quy et al. 2006; Pereira et al. 2005; Aguiar et al. 2009; Espinal et al. 2001; Suchindran et al. 2009), recent literature indicates an alarmingly high burden of drug-resistant TB among HIV-infected individuals (Isaakidis et al. 2014; Rajasekaran et al. 2009), with a significantly higher mortality rate and shorter survival period (Wells et al. 2007; Gandhi et al. 2006; Samuel et al. 2018). Several factors such as increased susceptibility to TB, malabsorption of anti-TB drugs resulting in suboptimal therapeutic blood levels, and interference of certain anti-TB drugs with antiretroviral drugs potentially increase the risk of MDR-TB in persons with HIV/AIDS. These data highlight the need to screen all chronic TB patients for TB drug resistance as well as HIV coinfection especially in HIV high prevalence settings.

Natural History of TB in People with HIV

Unlike most opportunistic infections which occur when the CD4+ T cell count drops down to 200 cells/mm^3, TB can occur at any point during the course of HIV disease (Havlir and Barnes 1999). HIV not only increases susceptibility to infection with *M. tuberculosis* but also increases the risk of progression of MTB infection to active TB disease (Getahun et al. 2010; Pawlowski et al. 2012). This risk increases with decrease in CD4+ T cell counts and worsening of the immune status (Diedrich and Flynn 2011). HIV-infected individuals usually become ill with active TB within weeks to months as a result of the underlying damage to their immune system, unlike in HIV negative individuals where the latency phase extends for several years, and in most cases over the lifetime.

Clinical Presentation of TB in HIV-Infected Individuals

The clinical presentation of TB in HIV-infected individuals depends on the degree of immunosuppression. In HIV-infected persons with a relatively intact immune system, pulmonary TB is the commonest form of TB (Burman and Jones 2003). In these individuals the chest radiographic findings are similar to those seen in HIV negative pulmonary TB cases with upper lobe infiltrates and cavitation, and sputum smears are often positive for acid-fast bacilli (Padyana et al. 2012). However, in those with advanced immunosuppression, extrapulmonary disease is more common. About 40–80% of HIV-infected people with TB are reported to develop extrapulmonary disease as compared to 10–20% among people without HIV (Sterling 2010). The commonest forms of extrapulmonary TB include pleural effusion, lymphadenopathy, pericardial disease, military disease, meningitis, and disseminated TB (WHO 2004). In those with pulmonary TB, chest radiographic findings resemble that of bacterial pneumonia with absence of cavities (Perlman et al. 1997). Sputum smears are seldom positive for acid-fast bacilli. In addition, up to one-fifth of the individuals with both pulmonary TB and HIV infection have normal chest X-rays (Greenberg et al. 1994).

As in adults, the natural history of TB in a child infected with HIV depends on the stage of HIV disease. Early in HIV infection, when the immunity is good, the signs of TB are similar to those in a child without HIV infection. As HIV infection progresses and immunity declines, dissemination of TB becomes more common. Tuberculous meningitis, military TB, and widespread tuberculous lymphadenopathy occur.

Diagnosis of TB in Persons Coinfected with HIV

The WHO estimated that 57% of TB cases among people living with HIV were not diagnosed or treated, resulting in 390,000 tuberculosis-related deaths among people living with HIV in 2015 (WHO 2016). This is because diagnosis of active TB disease in HIV-infected persons is much more challenging than in HIV uninfected individuals. Symptom-based screening for TB has limited utility in establishing a diagnosis in HIV positive individuals as they often do not manifest typical symptoms of TB. HIV infection compromises the effectiveness of chest X-ray in the diagnosis of pulmonary TB in HIV-infected persons. A significant proportion of HIV-infected persons who have culture-confirmed pulmonary TB have normal chest X-rays (Yoo et al. 2011). A large proportion of TB/HIV coinfected individuals (24–61%) are sputum smear negative because they are less likely to have cavitary lesions due to the impaired granuloma formation (Palmieri et al. 2002; Getahun et al. 2007; Dembele et al. 2008). Mycobacterial culture in liquid medium is much more sensitive than smear microscopy and is routinely recommended to aid in the diagnosis of TB in HIV-infected individuals (Gil-Setas et al. 2004; Lee et al. 2003; WHO 2007).

Higher rate of extrapulmonary disease offers another major challenge to the diagnosis of TB among HIV-infected individuals. Over the last decade, nucleic acid amplification tests (NAATs) that can amplify nucleic acid regions specific for *M. tuberculosis* and can be used directly on clinical samples have been developed (Vittor et al. 2014). NAATs yield results rapidly and are highly specific with improved sensitivity. These techniques can also detect specific mutations, thus providing information on drug sensitivity as well. The use of Xpert MTB/RIF (GeneXpert), a cartridge-based, TB-specific, nucleic acid amplification assay that can identify the presence of *M. tuberculosis* and mutations associated with rifampicin (RIF) resistance within 2 h, has increased significantly worldwide for the detection of paucibacillary forms of TB. The WHO endorsed Xpert MTB/RIF (Cepheid Inc., CA, USA) in December 2010 (WHO 2011a) and recommended the use of this assay since 2013 as the diagnostic test in adults and children suspected of having HIV-associated TB or multidrug-resistant TB (WHO 2013a). The Xpert MTB/RIF test has a pooled sensitivity of 88% and specificity of 99% when used as the initial diagnostic test instead of smear microscopy (Dorman et al. 2018). However, the pooled sensitivity of the test decreases to 79% in HIV-infected patients. Xpert-Ultra is an improved version that can detect *M. tuberculosis* infection as well as rifampicin resistance even among smear negative patients with HIV where the conventional Xpert MTB/RIF has a lesser yield (Chakravorty et al. 2017).

Loop-mediated isothermal amplification and fluorescence in situ hybridization using peptide nucleic acid probes are other rapid and simplified molecular techniques using NAAT platform to diagnose Mycobacterial infection, with high sensitivity and specificity (Boehme et al. 2007; Hongmanee et al. 2001). Lawn (2012) demonstrated that use of urine instead of sputum for Xpert MTB/RIF testing results in diagnosis of more cases of TB in HIV coinfected patients, indicating the value of urine samples for diagnosis of TB in these individuals. Other molecular tests, including MTBDRplus and LightCycler Mycobacterium Detection, have demonstrated specificities of more than 97%, but the sensitivity is reduced by 6% when compared with Xpert MTB/RIF test in HIV-infected patients with pulmonary TB (Scott et al. 2011).

Another promising molecular TB diagnostic test is detection of structural MTB-specific molecules such as lipoarabinomannan (LAM), a component of the cell wall of MTB that may be found in urine of patients with active TB (Sakamuri et al. 2013). The WHO recommended this method for diagnosis of HIV-associated TB in patients with very low CD4 cell counts (<100 cells/mm^3) and advanced immunodeficiency (WHO 2015a). Interestingly, a study from Shah et al. (2016) reported that combining urine LAM assay with Xpert MTB/RIF testing of urine could be an important opportunity to improve the diagnosis of active TB in HIV coinfected patients. Biomarkers measurable in the urine are of particular interest in the HIV-infected population, because they represent an easy, quick, and inexpensive method that can be used in diagnostic laboratories for TB diagnosis, and overcome the critical challenge of collecting enough sputum samples from HIV patients with advanced immunodeficiency. The new generation of molecular diagnostic tests is oriented toward the integration of TB and HIV diagnosis (Mendez-Samperio 2017).

Treatment of HIV-TB Coinfection

Treatment of patients with HIV-TB coinfection has improved over the years, attributable to improvements in antiretroviral and anti-tuberculosis treatment (ATT). HIV-infected individuals are prescribed the same regimen and course of daily dosing of TB drugs as HIV-uninfected TB patients. Currently, a 2-month initial intensive phase of isoniazid, rifampin, pyrazinamide, and ethambutol followed by

4 months of continuation phase of isoniazid and rifampin is considered as the standard treatment regimen for drug-susceptible TB. The Centres for Disease Control, Atlanta, recommends extension of ATT beyond 6 months in HIV coinfected pulmonary TB patients in specific instances like delayed sputum conversion, poor clinical prognosis, low CD4 count at nadir, and presence of cavitations (CDC 2009).

A number of studies showed significantly lower cure rates, higher mortality and recurrence rates of TB after standard ATT in HIV coinfected patients as compared to HIV negative individuals (Ruiz-Navarro et al. 2005; Chaisson et al. 1996; Morris et al. 2003; Kwan and Ernst 2011; Bell and Noursadeghi 2018), indicating that treatment of TB alone in HIV-TB coinfected patients was not sufficient as it did not significantly increase the CD4 count or reduce the viral load in these individuals (Morris et al. 2003). ART reduced TB risk among HIV-1-infected people by 54–90% and halved TB recurrence rate (Lawn and Meintjes 2011). This prompted the WHO to recommend ART initiation irrespective of CD4 count in HIV-TB coinfected individuals (WHO 2009a, b). However, this can be quite challenging due to potential drug-drug interactions, overlapping toxicities, difficulty adhering to medications, and an increased risk for immune reconstitution inflammatory syndrome (IRIS) (Egelund et al. 2017).

Early initiation of ART has been shown to not only reduce mortality and morbidity due to HIV and TB but also contribute to faster sputum conversion and prevent secondary complications like IRIS. Several studies have examined the appropriate timing for initiation of ART, and the findings reveal that early initiation of ART significantly improved survival of HIV-infected patients with TB (Török et al. 2011; Blanc et al. 2011; Abdool Karim et al. 2010; Havlir et al. 2011; Manosuthi et al. 2012; Uthman et al. 2015; Mfinanga et al. 2014; Abay et al. 2015). The current World Health Organization guidelines recommend that ART should be started as soon as possible "within the first 8 weeks" of starting anti-TB treatment and within the first 2 weeks for patients who have CD4 cell counts <50 cells/mm^3 (WHO 2012, 2013b, 2015b). Non-nucleoside reverse transcriptase inhibitor (NNRTI)-based ART remains the first-line regimen for HIV-infected patients with TB in most resource-limited settings. Although a standard dose of both efavirenz and nevirapine can be used, efavirenz is preferred because substantial pharmacokinetic interactions have been reported between rifampicin, a key component of anti-tuberculosis treatment, and antiretroviral drugs belonging to the NNRTI, Protease inhibitor and Integrase inhibitor classes. Tenofovir, emtricitabine/lamivudine along with efavirenz as a single pill once a day is the most recommended (Department of Health and Human Services 2016).

Non-rifampicin regimens in HIV have been associated with inferior outcomes (O'Donnel et al. 2002). Among the rifamycins, rifabutin induces hepatic cytochrome CYP3A4 the least and is the preferred rifamycin for concurrent administration with HAART (Regazzi et al. 2014). In resource-limited settings where rifabutin is not available, ritonavir-boosted saquinavir (SQV/r) is the recommended PI, and efavirenz at increased dosage (800 mg/day) is the preferred NNRTI to be given along with two NRTIs, for concurrent administration with rifampicin containing anti-tuberculosis regimens (Maartens et al. 2009).

Adverse reactions to either anti-TB or antiretroviral drugs as well IRIS are common in patients receiving integrated therapy than among TB patients without HIV (serious ADR—27 vs 13%), occurring mostly in the first 2 months of treatment (Yimer et al. 2008). Hepatoxicity is common due to shared metabolic pathways of anti-TB and antiretroviral drugs (Pukenyte et al. 2007; Narendran et al. 2013). Early recognition and appropriate management of these conditions is very important for treatment success. Many countries are moving toward the establishment of integrated healthcare facilities for TB and HIV, to offer holistic evaluation of those with both diseases, and practical management when patients encounter adverse drug effects.

Prognosis of MDR-TB in HIV continues to be grave with a death rate of over 50% (Palacios et al. 2012). Similarly, optimal treatment options for HIV/TB coinfected children are limited. It is important to undertake treatment studies in these crucial areas of research.

Tuberculosis Immune Reconstitution Inflammatory Syndrome (TB-IRIS)

Tuberculosis immune reconstitution inflammatory syndrome (TB-IRIS) refers to the condition where there is a paradoxical worsening of the signs and symptoms after starting ART in those dually infected with TB and HIV, despite good immunological recovery and effective virological suppression. Most cases of IRIS occur within the first 3 months of starting ART (Manabe et al. 2007). Various studies have reported incidence rates ranging from 8% to 43% (Breton et al. 2004). Functional restoration of immune system (i.e., CD4+ T cells) causing a cytokine outburst with an overriding Th1 response is thought to be the primary mechanism for development of IRIS (Bourgarit et al. 2006). The most consistent risk factors for development of TB-IRIS are very low CD4+ T cell count, CD4/CD8 ratio, hemoglobin, weight, presence of disseminated disease, shorter ATT-ART time interval, extra pulmonary foci and other opportunistic infections at the time of ART initiation (Lawn and Meintjes 2011; Narendran et al. 2013; Gopalan et al. 2014). Interleukin-6, CRP, Interferon gamma (IFN-γ), sCD14, baseline levels of vitamin D and higher D-dimer have been identified as predictors for risk of IRIS (Musselwhite et al. 2016). Fever with rigor or chills is the commonest and consistent symptom of TB-IRIS, with lymph node enlargement being the commonest manifestation (Breton et al. 2004). Anti-inflammatory drugs, especially steroids, form the backbone therapy for TB-IRIS (Meintjes et al. 2010). ART initiation before CD4 goes down considerably could protect against opportunistic infections and subsequent IRIS. In addition to ART, another intervention that decreases the risk of TB in HIV-infected patients is isoniazid preventive therapy, which reduces TB risk by 32% in ART-naive people and 37% in those on ART (The TEMPRANO ANRS 12136 Study Group 2015).

Isoniazid Preventive Therapy (IPT) for HIV-Infected Individuals

Mortality within the first 6 months after initiating ART has been attributed to TB in most resource-limited settings. Synergistic protection, with greater than 50% reduction in TB rates, was found in those who received both IPT and ART, than those who received either treatment alone (Rangaka et al. 2012). In 2011, the WHO released simplified guidelines for IPT, using the clinical algorithm of any cough, night sweats, weight loss, and/or fever, as well as household contact with sputum smear positive pulmonary TB cases, especially children for screening for TB and delivery of IPT (WHO 2011b).

Immune Response to *M. tuberculosis* Infection

M. tuberculosis infection begins through inhalation of air droplets containing the bacilli. The bacilli are rapidly phagocytosed by resident macrophages in the alveoli. Phagocytosis of *M. tuberculosis* by macrophages induces a state of cellular activation mediated by the production of a host of proinflammatory cytokines, followed by development of granuloma, which prevents dissemination of the pathogen and spread of disease. Cell-mediated immune responses mediated by CD4+ T lymphocytes play an important role in the prevention of subsequent disease progression.

Aberration of Innate Immune Responses in HIV-Infected Individuals

In HIV-infected individuals, a small proportion of the alveolar macrophages are also infected with the virus. Infected macrophages are defective in innate immune responses like phagocytosis (Jambo et al. 2014), antigen presentation (Leeansyah et al. 2007), and elimination of intracellular pathogens (Patel et al. 2007). HIV-infected macrophages have been shown to undergo less apoptosis in response to *M. tuberculosis* than uninfected macrophages (Patel et al. 2007). HIV can also infect and manipulate dendritic cell (DC) functions (Donaghy et al. 2004) and facilitate transmission and immune escape of both *M. tuberculosis* and HIV (van Kooyk et al. 2003). Migration of infected DCs also contributes to pathogen dissemination. Binding of mycobacterial ManLAM to DC-SIGN (dendritic cell-specific intercellular-adhesion-molecule-3-grabbing non-integrin) has been shown to inhibit DC maturation, increase IL-10 production, and decrease IL-12 production in response to lipopolysaccharides (Geijtenbeek et al. 2003; Nigou et al. 2001), which can hamper the initiation of a protective adaptive immune response against *M. tuberculosis*.

Elevated peripheral blood neutrophil count has been reported to be independently associated with active pulmonary TB and *M. tuberculosis* burden in sputum of HIV-infected people and is an independent predictor of mortality in those with TB (Kerkhoff et al. 2013). However, little work has been done on the role of neutrophils in HIV-TB coinfection. Neutrophils from ART-naive HIV-infected individuals have been demonstrated to have reduced capability to control *M. tuberculosis* growth as compared to neutrophils from uninfected controls (Martineau et al. 2007). Natural Killer (NK) cells are also innate immune cells that mediate killing of target cells through the release of cytoplasmic granules containing granulysin, perforin, and granzymes. NK cells have been shown to contribute to the control of *M. tuberculosis* infection in monocytes and macrophage cultures in vitro through cytolysis and induction of apoptosis of infected cells (Vankayalapati et al. 2004; Brill et al. 2001). NK cells from HIV-infected persons have been demonstrated to have significantly diminished cytolytic function (Fogli et al. 2004).

Impaired Acquired Immune Responses in HIV-Infected Individuals

A hallmark of HIV infection is a quantitative decline in CD4+ T lymphocytes, as well as generalized impairment of T cell helper function (Munier and Kelleher 2007). HIV-1 mediates decline in CD4 count through multiple mechanisms including decreased production and maturation, increased destruction through direct cellular infection by the virus, and so-called bystander cell death in the absence of direct infection. Depletion of CD4+ T cells has been observed in the lungs as well as bronchoalveolar lavage of HIV-infected individuals with active pulmonary TB. Peripheral CD4 count has been shown to correlate inversely with TB risk, with CD4 counts of ≥ 300 cells/mm^3 associated with one-third lower risk of active TB during a 3–6 month follow-up as compared to those with CD4 counts ≤ 100 cells/mm^3 in HIV-1-infected persons on ART (Chang et al. 2015). Peripheral CD4 count also correlates inversely with bacterial burden in those infected with HIV and TB (Mondal and Mandal 2015; Rao et al. 2015).

Significantly impaired *M. tuberculosis*-specific T cell function has also been observed in T cells obtained from HIV-infected people (Kalsdorf et al. 2009; Jambo et al. 2011). MTB-specific T cells were found to be less mature and produced comparatively little MIP-1α and more IL-2 in those with dual infection (Geldmacher et al. 2010). HIV also affects antigen presentation. The frequency of programmed cell death protein 1 expression has been found to be increased on T cells producing IFN-γ in response to PPD stimulation in HIV-TB coinfected individuals as compared to IFN-γ-producing T cells from those with TB alone, LTBI and HIV-1 infection, or LTBI alone (Pollock et al. 2016).

Even in people on ART where CD4+ T cells are numerically reconstituted, there is still a significantly increased risk of tuberculosis. This is hypothesized either to be due to persistent impairment of the quality of CD4+ T cell responses to *M. tuberculosis* or because certain subsets of CD4+ T cells do not recover quantitatively, regardless of ART (Du Bruyn and Wilkinson 2016). As previously mentioned, functional impairment of MTB-specific CD4+ lymphocytes in HIV-1 infection plays a key role in coinfection with TB.

CD8+ T cells form an important component of the immune response to intracellular pathogens (Gulzar and Copeland 2004). They mediate killing of infected cells via secretion of granzymes and perforins and induce apoptosis by activating cell death receptors on target cells (Woodworth et al. 2008). CD8+ T cells from HIV-TB coinfected persons exhibit decreased expression of the degranulation marker CD107a and impaired proliferative capacity in response to ESAT-6/CFP-10 (Kalokhe et al. 2015). Further, CD8+ T cells from HIV and HIV-TB coinfected individuals had higher expression of programmed cell death protein 1 (PD-1), a marker of CD8 T cell dysfunction, than healthy controls (Barber et al. 2006).

Immune Activation in HIV-TB Coinfected Individuals

Chronic immune activation has been recognized as a characteristic feature of HIV infection. *M. tuberculosis* infection contributes to the immune activation in HIV-TB coinfected people, with this effect persisting beyond clinical cure of TB. The persistent immune activation is believed to accelerate progression to AIDS, and increase risk of concomitant opportunistic infection and death in these individuals (Paiardini and Muller-Trutwin 2013; Boulougoura and Sereti 2016). Active TB in HIV-1-coinfected individuals induces higher levels of soluble markers of activation (soluble CD14, IL-6, IL-8, neopterin, β2-microglobulin, soluble TNF-α receptor I, etc.) and T cell surface activation markers (CD38 and HLA-DR) (Hanna et al. 2009). Interestingly, coinfected individuals with latent TB also had increased levels of T cell, but not monocyte, activation (Sullivan et al. 2015).

Exacerbation of HIV Infection by *M. tuberculosis* Coinfection

M. tuberculosis has been reported to upregulate HIV-1 replication in chronically or acutely infected T cells and macrophages (Shattock et al. 1993; Zhang et al. 1995), as well as ex vivo in alveolar macrophages and lymphocytes from patients with HIV infection (Toossi et al. 1997; Goletti et al. 1998). These in vitro/ex vivo findings are also reflected in vivo in HIV-infected individuals with concomitant active TB disease (Goletti et al. 1996). Very often, a transient decrease in CD4+ T cell count and a 5–160-fold increase in viral load have been demonstrated during *M. tuberculosis* infection in those with HIV-1 infection (Havlir and Barnes 1999; Munsiff et al. 1998).

It has been suggested that *M. tuberculosis* infection generates a microenvironment that facilitates HIV infection and replication by increasing the expression of co-receptors, upregulating pro-inflammatory cytokine production, and downregulating CCL5 (Rosas-Taraco et al. 2006). In vitro studies have also demonstrated that MTB infection favors replication of CXCR4 HIV variants by upregulation of CXCR4 and increase the efficiency of virus transmission from infected monocyte-derived macrophages (MDMs) to T cells (Mancino et al. 1997). Both MTB and HIV stimulate release of TNF-α from infected cells. While TNF-α is required for control of bacterial growth, it is known to activate HIV replication in macrophages (Kedzierska et al. 2003), indicating that the host immune response initiated against one pathogen may promote the replication of another.

The full implications of enhanced viral replication at the site of TB disease are not fully understood, but the error-prone transcriptional process of HIV-1 replication has prompted investigation into a possible influence on HIV-1 heterogeneity in the host. In cases of active pulmonary TB, the degree of viral heterogeneity was found to be greater in *M. tuberculosis*-infected lung segments than in uninfected lung segments (Nakata et al. 1997). Collins et al. demonstrated that pulmonary TB in HIV-1-infected people resulted in a two- to threefold greater mutation frequency when compared to CD4 matched HIV-1 mono-infected persons (Collins et al. 2000). Further investigation is required to elucidate the repercussions of increased HIV-1 heterogeneity at the site of *M. tuberculosis* infection.

Conclusion

HIV complicates every aspect of pulmonary tuberculosis from diagnosis to treatment, demanding a different approach to effectively tackle both the diseases. In order to control these converging epidemics, it is important to diagnose infection early, initiate appropriate therapy for both infections, prevent transmission, and administer preventive therapy. The current guidelines by WHO to start antiretroviral therapy irrespective of CD4+ cell count based on benefits cited by recent trials could go a long way in preventing various complications caused by the deadly duo.

Ultimately, the most cost-effective way of combating the two diseases would be vaccination. The present TB vaccine, BCG, does not effectively prevent the most prevalent form of the disease, pulmonary TB in adults. Similarly, no effective, preventive HIV vaccine can be discerned on the horizon, although many vaccine candidates are being evaluated in clinical trials. One approach would be to construct a combined TB/HIV vaccine. The design of candidate vaccines is, however, a particularly difficult task since laboratory correlates of protection have not been defined for *M. tuberculosis* and HIV infections. Since both pathogens enter the host through mucosal surfaces, a combination vaccine given at mucosal sites would probably be optimal. However, for this, further research on the biology of concurrent *M. tuberculosis* and HIV infections is urgently needed, using in vitro systems, animal models, and clinical studies, as well as vaccine trials.

Thus, an integrated approach to the two diseases would lead to the identification of new therapies to overcome the rapidly increasing drug resistance seen in both diseases, as well as for vaccination.

References

Abay, S. M., Deribe, K., Reda, A. A., Biadgilign, S., Datiko, D., Assefa, T., Todd, M., & Deribew, A. (2015). The effect of early initiation of antiretroviral therapy in TB/HIV co infected patients: A systematic review and meta-analysis. *Journal of the International Association of Providers of AIDS Care, 14*(6), 560–570.

Abdool Karim, S. S., Naidoo, K., Grobler, A., Padayatchi, N., Baxter, C., Gray, A., et al. (2010). Timing of initiation of antiretroviral drugs during tuberculosis therapy. *The New England Journal of Medicine, 362*, 697–706.

Aguiar, F., Vieira, M. A., Staviack, A., et al. (2009). Prevalence of anti-tuberculosis drug resistance in an HIV/AIDS reference hospital in Rio de Janeiro, Brazil. *The International Journal of Tuberculosis and Lung Disease, 13*, 54–61.

Barber, D. L., Wherry, E. J., Masopust, D., Zhu, B., Allison, J. P., Sharpe, A. H., Freeman, G. J., & Ahmed, R. (2006). Restoring function in exhausted CD8 T cells during chronic viral infection. *Nature, 439*, 682–687.

Bell, L. C. K., & Noursadeghi, M. (2018). Pathogenesis of HIV-1 and Mycobacterium tuberculosis co-infection. *Nature Reviews. Microbiology, 16*, 80–90.

Blanc, F. X., Sok, T., Laureillard, D., Borand, L., Rekacewicz, C., Nerrienet, E., et al. (2011). Earlier versus later start of antiretroviral therapy in HIV-infected adults with tuberculosis. *The New England Journal of Medicine, 365*, 1471–1481.

Boehme, C. C., Nabeta, P., Henostroza, G., et al. (2007). Operational feasibility of using loop-mediated isothermal amplification for diagnosis of pulmonary tuberculosis in microscopy centres of developing countries. *Journal of Clinical Microbiology, 45*, 1936–1940.

Boulougoura, A., & Sereti, I. (2016). HIV infection and immune activation: the role of co infections. *Current Opinion in HIV and AIDS, 11*(2), 191–200.

Bourgarit, A., Carcelain, G., Martinez, V., et al. (2006). ExPLOS ion of tuberculin-specific Th1-responses induces immune restoration syndrome in tuberculosis and HIV co-infected patients. *AIDS, 20*(2), F1–F7.

Breton, G., Duval, X., Estellat, C., et al. (2004). Determinants of immune reconstitution inflammatory syndrome in HIV type 1-infected patients with tuberculosis after initiation of antiretroviral therapy. *Clinical Infectious Diseases, 39*(11), 1709–1712.

Brill, K. J., Li, Q., Larkin, R., Canaday, D. H., Kaplan, D. R., Boom, W. H., & Silver, R. F. (2001). Human natural killer cells mediate killing of intracellular Mycobacterium tuberculosis H37Rv via granule-independent mechanisms. *Infection and Immunity, 69*, 1755–1765.

Burman, W. J., & Jones, B. E. (2003). Clinical and radiographic features of HIV-related tuberculosis. *Seminars in Respiratory Infections, 18*, 262–271.

Centre for Disease Control. (2009). Guidelines for prevention and treatment of opportunistic infections in HIV-infected adults and adolescents. *American Thoracic Society MMWR, 58*, 1–198.

Chaisson, R. E., Clermont, H. C., Holt, E. A., et al. (1996). Six-month supervised intermittent tuberculosis therapy in Haitian patients with and without HIV. *American Journal of Respiratory and Critical Care Medicine, 154*, 1034–1038.

Chakravorty, S., Simmons, A. M., Rowneki, M., Parmar, H., Cao, Y., Ryan, J., Banada, P. P., Deshpande, S., Shenai, S., Gall, A., Glass, J., Krieswirth, B., Schumacher, S. G., Nabeta, P., Tukvadze, N., Rodrigues, C., Skrahina, A., Tagliani, E., Cirillo, D. M., Davidow, A., Denkinger, C. M., Persing, D., Kwiatkowski, R., Jones, M., & Alland, D. (2017). The new Xpert MTB/RIF Ultra: Improving detection of Mycobacterium tuberculosis and resistance to rifampin in an assay suitable for point-of-care testing. *MBio, 8*(4), e00812–e00817.

Chang, C. A., Meloni, S. T., Eisen, G., Chaplin, B., Akande, P., Okonkwo, P., Rawizza, H. E., Tchetgen Tchetgen, E., & Kanki, P. J. (2015). Tuberculosis incidence and risk factors among human immunodeficiency virus (HIV)-infected adults receiving antiretroviral therapy in a large HIV program in Nigeria. *Open Forum Infectious Diseases, 2*, ofv154.

Chum, H. J., O'Brien, R. J., Chonde, T. M., Graf, P., & Rieder, H. L. (1996). An epidemiological study of tuberculosis and HIV infection in Tanzania, 1991–1993. *AIDS, 10*, 299–309.

Collins, K. R., Mayanja-Kizza, H., Sullivan, B. A., Quiñones-Mateu, M. E., Toossi, Z., & Arts, E. J. (2000). Greater diversity of HIV-1 quasispecies in HIV-infected individuals with active tuberculosis. *Journal of Acquired Immune Deficiency Syndromes, 24*, 408–417.

Dembele, M., Saleri, N., Migliori, G. B., Ouedraogo, H., Carvalho, A. C., Ouedraogo, M., et al. (2008). High incidence of sputum smear negative tuberculosis during HAART in Burkina Faso. *The European Respiratory Journal, 32*, 1668–1669.

Department of Health and Human Services. (2016). *Panel on antiretroviral guidelines for adults and adolescents.* http://www.aidsinfo.nih.gov/ContentFiles/AdultandAdolescentGL.pdf.

Diedrich, C. R., & Flynn, J. L. (2011). HIV-Mycobacterium tuberculosis coinfection immunology: How does HIV-1 exacerbate tuberculosis? *Infection and Immunity, 79*(4), 1407–1417.

Donaghy, H., Stebbing, J., & Patterson, S. (2004). Antigen presentation and the role of dendritic cells in HIV. *Current Opinion in Infectious Diseases, 17*, 1–6.

Dorman, S. E., Schumacher, S. G., Alland, D., Nabeta, P., Armstrong, D. T., King, B., Hall, S. L., Charavorty, S., Cirillo, D. M., Tukvadze, N., Bablishvili, N., Stevens, W., Scott, L., Rodrigues, C., Kazi, M. I., Joloba, M., Nakiyingi, L., Nocol, M. P., Ghebrekristos, Y., Anyango, I., Murithi, W., Dietze, R., Peres, R. L., Skrahina, A., Auchynka, V., Chopra, K. K., Hanif, M., Liu, X., Yuan, X., Boehme, C. C., Ellner, J. J., & Denkinger, C. M. (2018). Xpert MTB/RIF Ultra for detection of Mycobacterium tuberculosisand rifampicin resistance: A prospective multicentre diagnostic accuracy study. *The Lancet Infectious Diseases, 18*(1), 76–84.

Du Bruyn, E., & Wilkinson, R. J. (2016). The immune interaction between HIV-1 infection and Mycobacterium tuberculosis. *Microbiology Spectrum, 4*(6): TBTB2-0012-2016.

Egelund, E. F., Dupree, L., Huesgen, E., & Peloquin, C. A. (2017). The pharmacological challenges of treating tuberculosis and HIV coinfections. *Expert Review of Clinical Pharmacology, 10*(2), 213–223.

Espinal, M. A., Laserson, K., Camacho, M., et al. (2001). Determinants of drug-resistant tuberculosis: Analysis of 11 countries. *The International Journal of Tuberculosis and Lung Disease, 5*, 887–893.

Fogli, M., Costa, P., Murdaca, G., Setti, M., Mingari, M. C., Moretta, L., Moretta, A., & De Maria, A. (2004). Significant NK cell activation associated with decreased cytolytic function in peripheral blood of HIV-1-infected patients. *European Journal of Immunology, 34*, 2313–2321.

Gandhi, N. R., Moll, A., Sturm, A. W., et al. (2006). Extensively drug-resistant tuberculosis as a cause of death in patients co-infected with tuberculosis and HIV in a rural area of South Africa. *Lancet, 368*, 1575–1580.

Geijtenbeek, T. B., Van Vliet, S. J., Koppel, E. A., Sanchez-Hernandez, M., Vandenbroucke-Grauls, C. M., Appelmelk, B., & Van Kooyk, Y. (2003). Mycobacteria target DC-SIGN to suppress dendritic cell function. *The Journal of Experimental Medicine, 197*, 7–17.

Geldmacher, C., Ngwenyama, N., Schuetz, A., Petrovas, C., Reither, K., Heeregrave, E. J., Casazza, J. P., Ambrozak, D. R., Louder, M., Ampofo, W., Pollakis, G., Hill, B., Sanga, E., Saathoff, E., Maboko, L., Roederer, M., Paxton, W. A., Hoelscher, M., & Koup, R. A. (2010). Preferential infection and depletion of Mycobacterium tuberculosis-specific CD4 T cells after HIV-1 infection. *The Journal of Experimental Medicine, 207*, 2869–2881.

Getahun, H., Harrington, M., O'Brien, R., et al. (2007). Diagnosis of smear-negative pulmonary tuberculosis in people with HIV infection of AIDS in resource-constrained settings: Informing urgent policy changes. *Lancet, 369*, 2042–2049.

Getahun, H., Gunneberg, C., Granich, R., & Nunn, P. (2010). HIV infection-associated tuberculosis: The epidemiology and the response. *Clinical Infectious Diseases, 50*(Suppl 3), S201–S207.

Gil-Setas, A., Torroba, L., Fernandez, J. L., Martinez-Artola, V., & Olite, J. (2004). Evaluation of the MB/BacT system compared with Middlebrook 7H11 and Lowenstein-Jensen media for detection and recovery of mycobacteria from clinical specimens. *Clinical Microbiology and Infection, 10*, 224–228.

Goletti, D., Weissman, D., Jackson, R. W., Graham, N. M., Vlahov, D., et al. (1996). Effect of Mycobacterium tuberculosis on HIV replication: Role of immune activation. *Journal of Immunology, 157*, 1271–1278.

Goletti, D., Weissman, D., Jackson, R. W., Collins, F., Kinter, A., et al. (1998). The in vitro induction of human immunodeficiency virus (HIV) replication in purified protein derivative-positive HIV-infected persons by recall antigen response to Mycobacterium tuberculosis is the result of a balance of the effects of endogenous interleukin-2 and proinflammatory and antiinflammatory cytokines. *The Journal of Infectious Diseases, 177*, 1332–1338.

Gopalan, N., Andrade, B. B., & Swaminathan, S. (2014). Tuberculosis-immune reconstitution inflammatory syndrome in HIV: From pathogenesis to prediction. *Expert Review of Clinical Immunology, 10*(5), 631–645.

Greenberg, S. D., Frager, D., Suster, B., Walker, S., Stavropoulos, C., & Rothpearl, A. (1994). Active pulmonary tuberculosis in patients with AIDS: Spectrum of radiographic findings (including a normal appearance). *Radiology, 193*, 115–119.

Gulzar, N., & Copeland, K. F. (2004). CD8+ T-cells: Function and response to HIV infection. *Current HIV Research, 2*, 23–37.

Hanna, L. E., Nayak, K., Subramanyam, S., Venkatesan, P., Narayanan, P. R., & Swaminathan, S. (2009). Incomplete immunological recovery following anti-tuberculosis treatment in HIV-infected individuals with active tuberculosis. *The Indian Journal of Medical Research, 129*, 548–554.

Havlir, D. V., & Barnes, P. F. (1999). Tuberculosis in patients with human immunodeficiency virus infection. *The New England Journal of Medicine, 340*, 367–373.

Havlir, D. V., Kendall, M. A., Ive, P., Kumwenda, J., Swindells, S., Qasba, S. S., et al. (2011). Timing of antiretroviral therapy for HIV-1 infection and tuberculosis. *The New England Journal of Medicine, 365*, 1482–1491.

Hongmanee, P., Stender, H., & Rasmussen, O. F. (2001). Evaluation of a fluorescence in situ hybridization assay for differentiation between tuberculous and non-tuberculous mycobacteria species in smears of Lowenstein-Jensen and mycobacteria growth indicator tube cultures using peptide nucleic acid probes. *Journal of Clinical Microbiology, 39*, 1032–1035.

Isaakidis, P., Das, M., Kumar, A. M. V., Peskett, C., Khetarpal, M., Bamne, A., Adsul, B., Manglani, M., Sachdeva, K. S., Parmar, M., Kanchar, A., Rewari, B. B., Deshpande, A., Rodrigues, C., Shetty, A., Rebello, L., Saranchuk, P., Tyagi, A. K. (2014). Alarming levels of drug-resistant tuberculosis in HIV-infected patients in petropolitan Mumbai, India. *PLoS One, 9*(10), e110461.

Jambo, K. C., Sepako, E., Fullerton, D. G., Mzinza, D., Glennie, S., Wright, A. K., Heyderman, R. S., & Gordon, S. B. (2011). Bronchoalveolar CD4+ T cell responses to respiratory antigens are impaired in HIV-infected adults. *Thorax, 66*, 375–382.

Jambo, K. C., Banda, D. H., Kankwatira, A. M., Sukumar, N., Allain, T. J., Heyderman, R. S., Russell, D. G., & Mwandumba, H. C. (2014). Small alveolar macrophages are infected preferentially by HIV and exhibit impaired phagocytic function. *Mucosal Immunology, 7*, 1116–1126.

Kalokhe, A. S., Adekambi, T., Ibegbu, C. C., Ray, S. M., Day, C. L., & Rengarajan, J. (2015). Impaired degranulation and proliferative capacity of Mycobacterium tuberculosis-specific CD8+ T cells in HIV-infected individuals with latent tuberculosis. *The Journal of Infectious Diseases, 211*, 635–640.

Kalsdorf, B., Scriba, T. J., Wood, K., Day, C. L., Dheda, K., Dawson, R., Hanekom, W. A., Lange, C., & Wilkinson, R. J. (2009). HIV-1 infection impairs the bronchoalveolar T-cell response to mycobacteria. *American Journal of Respiratory and Critical Care Medicine, 180*, 1262–1270.

Kedzierska, K., Crowe, S. M., Turville, S., & Cunningham, A. L. (2003). The influence of cytokines, chemokines and their receptors on HIV-1 replication in monocytes and macrophages. *Reviews in Medical Virology, 13*, 39–56.

Kenyon, T. A., Mwasekaga, M. J., Huebner, R., Rumisha, D., Binkin, N., & Maganu, E. (1999). Low levels of drug resistance amidst rapidly increasing tuberculosis and human immunodeficiency virus co-epidemics in Botswana. *The International Journal of Tuberculosis and Lung Disease, 3*, 4–11.

Kerkhoff, A. D., Wood, R., Lowe, D. M., Vogt, M., & Lawn, S. D. (2013). Blood neutrophil counts in HIV-infected patients with pulmonary tuberculosis: Association with sputum mycobacterial load. *PLoS One, 8*(7), e67956.

Kwan, C. K., & Ernst, J. D. (2011). HIV and tuberculosis: A deadly human syndemic. *Clinical Microbiology Reviews, 24*, 351–376.

Lawn, S. D. (2012) Point-of-care detection of lipoarabinomannan (LAM) in urine for diagnosis of HIV-associated tuberculosis: a state of the art review. *BMC Infectious Diseases, 12*, 103

Lawn, S. D., & Meintjes, G. (2011). Pathogenesis and prevention of immune reconstitution disease during antiretroviral therapy. *Expert Review of Anti-Infective Therapy, 9*(4), 415–430.

Lee, J. J., Suo, J., Lin, C. B., Wang, J. D., Lin, T. Y., & Tsai, Y. C. (2003). Comparative evaluation of the BACTEC MGIT 960 system with solid medium for isolation of mycobacteria. *The International Journal of Tuberculosis and Lung Disease, 7*, 569–574.

Leeansyah, E., Wines, B. D., Crowe, S. M., & Jaworowski, A. (2007). The mechanism underlying defective Fcgamma receptor-mediated phagocytosis by HIV-1-infected human monocyte-derived macrophages. *Journal of Immunology, 178*, 1096–1104.

Maartens, G., Decloedt, E., & Cohen, K. (2009). Effectiveness and safety of antiretroviral with rifampicin: Crucial issues for high burden countries. *Antiviral Therapy, 14*, 1039–1043.

Manabe, Y. C., Campbell, J. D., Sydnor, E., et al. (2007). Immune reconstitution inflammatory syndrome: Risk factors and treatment implications. *Journal of Acquired Immune Deficiency Syndromes, 46*(4), 456–462.

Mancino, G., Placido, R., Bach, S., Mariani, F., Montesano, C., et al. (1997). Infection of human monocytes with Mycobacterium tuberculosis enhances human immunodeficiency virus type 1 replication and transmission to T cells. *The Journal of Infectious Diseases, 175*, 1531–1535.

Manosuthi, W., Mankatitham, W., Lueangniyomkul, A., Thongyen, S., Likanonsakul, S., Suwanvattana, P., et al. (2012). Time to initiate antiretroviral therapy between 4 weeks and 12 weeks of tuberculosis treatment in HIV-infected patients: Results from the TIME study. *Journal of Acquired Immune Deficiency Syndromes, 60*, 377–383.

Martineau, A. R., Newton, S. M., Wilkinson, K. A., Kampmann, B., Hall, B. M., Nawroly, N., Packe, G. E., Davidson, R. N., Griffiths, C. J., & Wilkinson, R. J. (2007). Neutrophil-mediated innate immune resistance to mycobacteria. *Journal of Clinical Investigation, 117*(7), 1988–1994.

Meintjes, G., Wilkinson, R. J., Morroni, C., et al. (2010). Randomized placebo-controlled trial of prednisone for paradoxical tuberculosis-associated immune reconstitution inflammatory syndrome. *AIDS, 24*(15), 2381–2390.

Mendez-Samperio, P. (2017). Diagnosis of tuberculosis in HIV co-infected individuals: Current status, challenges and opportunities for the future. *Scandinavian Journal of Immunology, 86*(2), 76–82.

Mfinanga, S. G., Kirenga, B. J., Chanda, D. M., Mutayoba, B., Mthiyane, T., Yimer, G., et al. (2014). Early versus delayed initiation of highly active antiretroviral therapy for HIV-positive adults with newly diagnosed pulmonary tuberculosis (TB-HAART): A prospective, international, randomised, placebo-controlled trial. *The Lancet Infectious Diseases, 14*, 563–571.

Mondal, K., & Mandal, R. (2015). Cytopathological and microbiological profile of tuberculous lymphadenitis in HIV-infected patients with special emphasis on its corroboration with CD4+ T-cell counts. *Acta Cytologica, 59*, 156–162.

Morris, L., Martin, D. J., Bredell, H., et al. (2003). HIV-1 RNA levels and CD4 lymphocyte counts during treatment for active tuberculosis in South African patients. *The Journal of Infectious Diseases, 187*, 1967–1971.

Munier, M. L., & Kelleher, A. D. (2007). Acutely dysregulated, chronically disabled by the enemy within: T-cell responses to HIV-1 infection. *Immunology and Cell Biology, 85*, 6–15.

Munsiff, S. S., Alpert, P. L., Gourevitch, M. N., Chang, C. J., Klein, R. S., Chang, C. J., & Klein, R. S. (1998). A prospective study of tuberculosis and HIV disease progression. *Journal of Acquired Immune Deficiency Syndromes and Human Retrovirology, 19*, 361–366.

Musselwhite, L. W., Andrade, B. B., Ellenberg, S. S., et al. (2016). Vitamin D, d-dimer, interferon gamma, and sCD14 levels are independently associated with immune reconstitution inflammatory syndrome: A prospective, international study. *eBioMedicine, 4*, 115–123.

Nakata, K., Rom, W. N., Honda, Y., Condos, R., Kanegasaki, S., Cao, Y., & Weiden, M. (1997). Mycobacterium tuberculosis enhances human immunodeficiency virus-1 replication in the lung. *American Journal of Respiratory and Critical Care Medicine, 155*, 996–1003.

Narendran, G., Andrade, B. B., Porter, B. O., et al. (2013). Paradoxical tuberculosis immune reconstitution inflammatory syndrome (TB-IRIS) in HIV patients with culture confirmed pulmonary tuberculosis in India and the potential role of IL-6 in prediction. *PLoS One, 8*(5), 63541.

Nigou, J., Zelle-Rieser, C., Gilleron, M., Thurnher, M., & Puzo, G. (2001). Mannosylated lipoarabinomannans inhibit IL-12 production by human dendritic cells: Evidence for a negative signal delivered through the mannose receptor. *Journal of Immunology, 166*, 7477–7485.

O'Donnel, M. M., Souza Carvalho, S., et al. (2002). Poor response to tuberculosis treatment with regiments without rifampicin in immunosuppressed AIDS patients. *The Brazilian Journal of Infectious Diseases, 6*(6), 272–275.

Padyana, M., Bhat, R. V., Dinesha, M., & Nawaz, A. (2012). HIV-tuberculosis: A study of chest X-ray patterns in relation to CD4 count. *North American Journal of Medical Sciences, 4*(5), 221–225.

Paiardini, M., & Muller-Trutwin, M. (2013). HIV-associated chronic immune activation. *Immunological Reviews, 254*(1), 78–101.

Palacios, E., Franke, M., Muñoz, M., et al. (2012). HIV-positive patients treated for multidrug-resistant tuberculosis: Clinical outcomes in the HAART era. *The International Journal of Tuberculosis and Lung Disease, 16*(3), 348–354.

Palmieri, A., Girardi, E., Pellicelli, A. M., et al. (2002). Pulmonary tuberculosis in HIV-infected patients presenting with normal chest radiograph and negative sputum smear. *Infection, 30*, 68–74.

Patel, N. R., Zhu, J., Tachado, S. D., Zhang, J., Wan, Z., Saukkonen, J., & Koziel, H. (2007). HIV impairs TNF-alpha mediated macrophage apoptotic response to Mycobacterium tuberculosis. *Journal of Immunology, 179*, 6973–6980.

Pawlowski, A., Jansson, M., Skold, M., Rottenberg, M. E., & Kallenius, G. (2012). Tuberculosis and HIV co-infection. *PLoS Pathogens, 8*(2), e1002464.

Pereira, M., Tripathy, S., Inamdar, V., et al. (2005). Drug resistance pattern of Mycobacterium tuberculosis in seropositive and seronegative HIV-TB patients in Pune, India. *Indian Journal of Medical Research, 121*, 235–239.

Perlman, D. C., el-Sadr, W. M., Nelson, E. T., Matts, J. P., Telzak, E. E., Salomon, N., et al. (1997). Variation of chest radiographic patterns in pulmonary tuberculosis by degree of human immunodeficiency virus-related immunosuppression. The Terry Beirn Community Programs for Clinical Research on AIDS (CPCRA). The AIDS Clinical Trials Group (ACTG). *Clinical Infectious Diseases, 25*, 242–246.

Pollock, K. M., Montamat-Sicotte, D. J., Grass, L., Cooke, G. S., Kapembwa, M. S., Kon, O. M., Sampson, R. D., Taylor, G. P., & Lalvani, A. (2016). PD-1 expression and cytokine secretion profiles of Mycobacterium tuberculosis-specific CD4+ T-cell subsets: Potential correlates of containment in HIV-TB co-infection. *PLoS One, 11*, e0146905.

Pukenyte, E., Lescure, F. X., Rey, D., et al. (2007). Incidence of and risk factors for severe liver toxicity in HIV-infected patients on anti-tuberculosis treatment. *The International Journal of Tuberculosis and Lung Disease, 11*, 78–84.

Quy, H. T., Buu, T. N., Cobelens, F. G., Lan, N. T., Lambregts, C. S., & Borgdorff, M. W. (2006). Drug resistance among smear-positive tuberculosis patients in Ho Chi Minh City, Vietnam. *The International Journal of Tuberculosis and Lung Disease, 10*, 160–166.

Rajasekaran S., Chandrasekar C., Mahilmaran A., Kanakaraj K., Karthikeyan D. S. A., Suriakumar, J. (2009). HIV coinfection among multidrug resistant and extensively drug resistant tuberculosis patients–a trend. *Journal of Indian Medical Association, 107*(5), 281–286.

Rangaka, M. X., Boulle, A., Wilkinson, R. J., et al. (2012). Randomized controlled trial of isoniazid preventive therapy in HIV-infected persons on antiretroviral therapy. *Clinical Infectious Diseases, 55*(12), 1698–1706.

Rao, J. S., Kumari, S. J., & Kini, U. (2015). Correlation of CD4 counts with the FNAC patterns of tubercular lymphadenitis in patients with HIV: A cross sectional pilot study. *Diagnostic Cytopathology, 43*, 16–20.

Regazzi, M., Carvalho, A. C., Villani, P., & Matteelli, A. (2014). Treatment optimization in patients co-infected with Mycobacterium tuberculosis infections: Focus on drug-drug interactions with rifamycins. *Clinical Pharmacokinetics, 53*(6), 489.

Rosas-Taraco, A. G., Arce-Mendoza, A. Y., Caballero-Olin, G., & Salinas-Carmona, M. C. (2006). Mycobacterium tuberculosis upregulates coreceptors CCR5 and CXCR4 while HIV modulates CD14 favoring concurrent infection. *AIDS Research and Human Retroviruses, 22*, 45–51.

Ruiz-Navarro, M. D., Hernández Espinosa, J. A., Bleda Hernández, M. J., et al. (2005). Effects of HIV status and other variables on the outcome of tuberculosis treatment in Spain. *Archivos de Bronconeumología, 41*(7), 363–370.

Sakamuri, R. M., Price, D. N., Lee, M., et al. (2013). Association of lipoarabinomannan with high density lipoprotein in blood: Implications for diagnostics. *Tuberculosis, 93*, 301–307.

Samuel, J. P., Sood, A., Campbell, J. R., Khan, F. A., & Johnston, J. C. (2018). Comorbidities and treatment outcomes in multidrug resistant tuberculosis: A systematic review and meta-analysis. *Scientific Reports, 8*, 4980.

Scott, L. E., McCarthy, K., Gous, N., Nduna, M., van Rie, A., Sanne, I., Venter, W. F., Duse, A., & Stevens, W. (2011). Comparison of Xpert MTB/RIF with other nucleic acid technologies for diagnosing pulmonary tuberculosis in a high HIV prevalence setting: A prospective study. *PLoS Medicine, 8*(7), e1001061.

Shah, M., Hanrahan, C., Wang, Z. Y., et al. (2016). Lateral flow urine lipoarabinomannan for detecting active tuberculosis in HIV-positive adults. *Cochrane Database of Systematic Reviews, 5*, CD011420.

Shattock, R. J., Friedland, J. S., & Griffin, G. E. (1993). Modulation of HIV transcription in and release from human monocytic cells following phagocytosis of Mycobacterium tuberculosis. *Research in Virology, 144*, 7–12.

Sterling, T. (2010). HIV infection-related tuberculosis: Clinical manifestations and treatment. *Clinical Infectious Diseases, 50*(3), S223–S230.

Suchindran, S., Brouwer, E. S., & Van Rie, A. (2009). Is HIV infection a risk factor for multi-drug resistant tuberculosis? A systematic review. *PLoS One, 4*, e5561.

Sullivan, Z. A., Wong, E. B., Ndung'u, T., Kasprowicz, V. O., & Bishai, W. R. (2015). Latent and active tuberculosis infection increase immune activation in individuals co-infected with HIV. *eBioMedicine, 2*, 334–340.

The TEMPRANO ANRS 12136 Study Group. (2015). A trial of early antiretrovirals and preventive therapy in Africa. *The New England Journal of Medicine, 373*, 808–822.

Toossi, Z., Nicolacakis, K., Xia, L., Ferrari, N. A., & Rich, E. A. (1997). Activation of latent HIV-1 by Mycobacterium tuberculosis and its purified protein derivative in alveolar macrophages from HIV-infected individuals in vitro. *Journal of Acquired Immune Deficiency Syndromes and Human Retrovirology, 15*, 325–331.

Török, M. E., Yen, N. T., Chau, T. T., Mai, N. T., Phu, N. H., Mai, P. P., et al. (2011). Timing of initiation of antiretroviral therapy in human immunodeficiency virus (HIV)–associated tuberculous meningitis. *Clinical Infectious Diseases, 52*, 1374–1383.

Uthman, O. A., Okwundu, C., Gbenga, K., Volmink, J., Dowdy, D., Zumla, A., et al. (2015). Optimal timing of antiretroviral therapy initiation for HIV-infected adults with newly diagnosed pulmonary tuberculosis: A systematic review and meta-analysis. *Annals of Internal Medicine, 163*, 32–39.

van Kooyk, Y., Appelmelk, B., & Geijtenbeek, T. B. (2003). A fatal attraction: Mycobacterium tuberculosis and HIV-1 target DC-SIGN to escape immune surveillance. *Trends in Molecular Medicine, 9*, 153–159.

Vankayalapati, R., Klucar, P., Wizel, B., Weis, S. E., Samten, B., Safi, H., Shams, H., & Barnes, P. F. (2004). NK cells regulate CD8+ T cell effector function in response to an intracellular pathogen. *Journal of Immunology, 172*, 130–137.

Vittor, A. Y., Garland, J. M., & Gilman, R. H. (2014). Molecular diagnosis of TB in the HIV positive population. *Annals of Global Health, 80*(6), 476–485.

Wells, C. D., Cegielski, J. P., Nelson, L. J., et al. (2007). HIV infection and multidrug-resistant tuberculosis: The perfect storm. *The Journal of Infectious Diseases, 196*(Suppl 1), S86–S107.

WHO. (2004). *TB/HIV: a clinical manual, Harries A, Maher D, Graham S. WHO/HTM/TB/2004.329* (2nd ed.). Geneva: WHO.

WHO. (2007). *Improving the diagnosis and treatment of smear-negative pulmonary and extrapulmonary tuberculosis among adults and adolescents: Recommendations for HIV-prevalent and resource-constrained settings, WHO/HTM/T B/2007.379*. Geneva: WHO.

WHO. (2008). *Implementing the WHO Stop TB Strategy: A handbook for national tuberculosis control programmers* (p. 67). Geneva: WHO www.who.int/tb/publications/2008/.

WHO. (2009a). *Rapid advice: Antiretroviral therapy for HIV infection in adults and adolescents.* http://www.searo.who.int/LinkFiles/HIV-AIDS_Rapid_Advice_Adult_ ART_ Guidelines(web).pdf.

WHO. (2009b). *Global tuberculosis control: Surveillance, planning, financing, WHO report 2009.* Geneva: WHO.

WHO. (2011a). *Rapid implementation of the Xpert MTB/RIF diagnostic test: Technical and operational "how to" practical considerations, WHO/HTM/TB/2011.2*. Geneva: WHO.

WHO. (2011b). *Guidelines for intensified tuberculosis case-finding and isoniazid preventive therapy for people living with HIV in resource-constrained settings.* Geneva: World Health Organization http://whqlibdoc.who.int/publications/2011/9789241500708_eng.pdf.

WHO. (2012). *WHO policy on collaborative TB/HIV activities: Guidelines for national programmes and other stakeholders.* http://www.who.int/tb/publications/2012/tb_hiv_policy_ 9789241503006/en/.

WHO. (2013a). *Automated real-time nucleic acid amplification technology for rapid and simultaneous detection of tuberculosis and rifampin resistance: Xpert MTB/RIF system for the diagnosis of pulmonary and extrapulmonary TB in adults and children. Policy update.* Geneva, Switzerland: WHO.

WHO. (2013b). *Consolidated guidelines on the use of antiretroviral drugs for treating and preventing HIV infection: Recommendations for a public health approach.* http://www.who.int/hiv/pub/guidelines/arv2013/.

WHO. (2015a). *The use of lateral flow urine lipoarabinomannan assay (LF-LAM) for the diagnosis and screening of active tuberculosis in people living with HIV. Policy update.* Geneva, Switzerland: WHO.

WHO. (2015b). *WHO global tuberculosis report 2015.* Geneva: WHO http://apps.who.int/iris/bitstream/10665/44165/1/9789241547833_eng.pdf?ua=1&ua=1.

WHO. (2016). *WHO global tuberculosis report 2016.* Geneva: WHO http://www.who.int/tb/publications/global_report/en/.

WHO. (2017). *Global tuberculosis control 2017.* Geneva: WHO www.who.int/tb/publications/global_report/en/.

WHO. (2018). *Tuberculosis control*. Retrieved 14 March 2018 from http://www.who.int/trade/distance_learning/gpgh/gpgh3/en/index4.htm.

Woodworth, J. S., Wu, Y., & Behar, S. M. (2008). Mycobacterium tuberculosis-specific CD8+ T cells require perforin to kill target cells and provide protection in vivo. *Journal of Immunology, 181*, 8595–8603.

Yimer, G., Aderaye, G., Amogne, W., et al. (2008). Anti-tuberculosis therapy-induced hepatotoxicity among Ethiopian HIV-positive and negative patients. *PLoS One, 3*(3), e1809.

Yoo, S. D., Cattamanchi, A., den Boon, S., Worodria, W., Kisembo, H., Huang, L., & Davis, J. L. (2011). Clinical significance of normal chest radiographs among HIV-seropositive patients with suspected tuberculosis in Uganda. *Respirology, 16*(5), 836–841.

Zhang, Y., Nakata, K., Weiden, M., & Rom, W. N. (1995). Mycobacterium tuberculosis enhances human immunodeficiency virus-1 replication by transcriptional activation at the long terminal repeat. *The Journal of Clinical Investigation, 95*, 2324–2331.

Printed in the United States
By Bookmasters